VIKING NINJA

ELEMENTS

Kill Your Ego,
Challenge Your Discipline

By Erik Melland and Robinson Erhardt

Copyright © Viking Ninja, LLC 2018

Sign up for our newsletter to learn more about the Viking Ninja belting system, training, and events at VKNJA.com.

Check out Erik Melland on Instagram at @erikmelland. For more ideas and inspiration, follow @VKNJA.

FOR BRUCE LEE

CONTENTS

Foreword	1
Introduction	4
Viking	8
Exceed Your Limits	14
The Valknut	21
Viking Ninja	28
Warrior Spirit	34
Total Human Optimization	40
Kill Your Ego	47
The Steel Mace	52
Ninja	62
Like Water	68
Challenge Your Discipline	74
Yin and Yang	80

Bodyweight	87
Honor Your Dedication	94
The Vegvisir Compass	100
Martial Arts	106
The Viking Ninja Sigil	111
Immortality	117
Viking Ninja Chakra	123
Belting System	129
Brotherhood	134
Recovery	140
Flow (Mindful Mechanics)	145
Education	153
Unconventional Training	158
Viking Ship on the Water	164
Afterword	169

VIKING NINJA

ELEMENTS

Kill Your Ego,
Challenge Your Discipline

FOREWORD

Fitness has always been part of my life. At first it was subconscious, but eventually the hunger to harness my body tore its way out of me. As a young full-time musician I wasn't getting any healthier. All the bars, cigarettes, and late nights didn't help. I dropped those habits to get my life back. I knew a regular job wouldn't cut it if I was going to be serious, so I went to massage school, where I learned to approach the body with care and attention. That was the first step.

Eventually I realized the need to delve deeper into fitness, but it was a long time before I found the person to help me along that path: John Wolf, the Chief Fitness Officer at Onnit Labs. He led me to Scott Sonnon, who had a product called club bells. The system around them was totally disciplined. It was tactical, and by tactical I mean military. It centered around respect, discipline, and honor. I have a deep love for the military in my heart because they still hold those values dear. Nobody else in this world knows a thing about them, but they've come to form the foundation of Viking Ninja.

I believe we must be tested to exceed our limitations. The human body should not be left alone. To abandon our bodies is to abandon our souls. And we're lazy. We're prone to rot. I work out to challenge myself. It's become an addiction for me, and I don't want a break. I train for the adrenaline rush, but I stay responsible with volume and intensity so that I can continue to feed my addiction every day.

I teach for the pure satisfaction of helping someone live longer for their son, for their mother, whoever it is. Prolonging and bettering life, whatever the situation, is my goal. I'm not here to make you a meathead or a cardio freak. I'm here to help you sculpt the perfect body while providing your mind with the food necessary for optimization. As humans we will never evolve internally if we don't break those external barriers.

The outlet for all my energy, Viking Ninja, operates under the principles of discipline, structure, integration, and owning everything you do. It's not about saying, "Let's have fun, pump iron, and move irresponsibly just to take a few cool pictures."

My motto at the Viking Ninja gym is, "Kill your ego. Challenge your discipline." There's too much arrogance in fitness these days. Viking Ninja does not stand for that. We represent the martial arts philosophy that leads toward honoring your commitment by giving one hundred percent. This will enable you to move efficiently, grow stronger, live longer, and build an unbreakable nervous system.

If that's your goal, you have to strive. Once walls are knocked down you'll look back and think, "Wow, that took a long time. I'm sixty years old but I feel twenty." The most tragic thing in life is when people retire with all the money they've amassed but they're too broken to savor it. They've been crushed beneath the wheel. They didn't do any maintenance work. They can't enjoy the fruits of their labor because they failed their bodies. Achieving the opposite is the goal with Viking Ninja's education system. We want to discipline the fitness industry.

I built this because I always wanted something of my own. I had a unique way of training but I didn't know how to deliver it until I came to Onnit, where I was given an opportunity to express myself on their platform. I'm very grateful for that. At the same time, I created Viking Ninja not only to help people grow healthy and strong—those reasons are obvious—but so that I could continue sharing my training methods and philosophy with others. I want my friends and students to improve their lives because it means something to them—not just to pose for the cameras.

- Erik "Esik" Melland

INTRODUCTION

Esik is a genius. He understands the human body on an intuitive level that few people I've met come close to matching. Esik is also deeply philosophical, and none of the content in this book comes from me.

My contribution came in the form of sitting before a keyboard. I may have extreme finger endurance, but they don't give awards for that. What I've managed to cobble together here comes directly from Esik's mind, though he'll be the first person to tell you that he's the result of a long, storied lineage of thinkers and movers. After this section, the rest of the text's words belong to him.

Perhaps most directly influential to this book is Onnit, where Esik was first introduced to the steel mace. Onnit's mission is Total Human Optimization, which inspired the vision behind Viking Ninja: to better any and every person willing to give their all toward achieving that end. Without Onnit neither one of us would be where we are today.

The most significant individual character in Viking Ninja's origin story is one Esik never met: Bruce Lee. There are other players as well, Vikings and ninjas chief among them—and they haven't been around for hundreds of years. Even the Ninja Turtles had a role in the system's development. When Esik was a kid he wanted to be a Ninja Turtle more than anything else. Apparently nobody ever told him it wasn't possible, as he's come pretty close.

Our purpose here is to take the totality of Viking Ninja and distill it into easily accessible pieces. There's a lot of material in this book, but it barely scratches the surface of what's in Esik's head. The text is often dense, and to absorb it will require patience, time, and reflection.

I've broken everything down into twenty-six chapters, each of which covers a single element. They lead into one another and intermingle, but you can also skip around, though some things may not be wholly clear if you've missed earlier sections. If you come across something you don't like—maybe your ancestors were killed by ninjas and you still harbor resentment against them—feel free to skip it.

While some chapters are purely philosophical, others explain the reasoning behind physical aspects of the system—like the steel mace—and how they can contribute to anyone's development, regardless of whether you consider yourself an athlete. When taken as a whole, this book will give you a firm grounding in the values of Viking Ninja. Still, don't take anything written here as fact. Please disagree as much as possible. My only request is that you give everything careful consideration before you make judgment.

This project wasn't without its challenges for me. Esik speaks a completely different language from what I'm used to. If anything, my nature is to be mathematical, scientific, and precise. I spent a lot of time thinking about whether or not I should capitalize "ninja," if that tells you anything (and I've decided to do so only when it refers to the Esik's concept rather than the actual thing). If Esik makes an offhand comment about how some form of mace rotation improves shoulder mobility, I want to see studies in the literature that support him. Unfortunately I've had to accept that science often lags ten to twenty years behind what happens in the gym, and instead have had to rely upon my own experience, as well as that of people I trust.

At the beginning I had trouble relating to Esik's philosophy. I have a degree in the same, but not the Eastern, spiritual kind that Esik is so in tune with. My version of philosophy is rigorous and reads more like math than anything else, whereas Esik's taps deep into the human soul in search of higher knowledge and inspiration. Before writing this I preferred symbolic logic and strict reasoning. How do you prove some of Esik's arguments? You can't. What you have to do is look inside yourself and listen for an echo—do they resonate with the truest parts of your being?

Picture yourself walking into the modern wing of an art museum. Countless people—and I've certainly been one of them—see blank canvases with a few splotches on them and scoff. That's judgment, and the opposite of open-mindedness. Much as with learning about Viking Ninja, I once went on an art history binge and realized that the beauty wasn't necessarily in the paint on the canvas, but in the ideas and emotions conveyed by the artist. Jackson Pollock, for example, turned art on its head by rejecting conventions and becoming a god of the canvas, no longer limited by anything so obvious as form or material.

As with art, it all comes down to interpretation. There are many images and symbols in this book central to Viking Ninja, and which we evaluate and ascribe meaning to much as one might a painting in that same modern art wing. There aren't "right" or "wrong" interpretations—what matters is how they sit with you and in turn benefit your life.

Two crossed planks of wood can mean a lot of things, but for billions of people in the world they form a symbol that makes life under even the most arduous conditions bearable and worthwhile. There's no reason a steel mace and a shield can't do the same. You are the one who gives every chapter purpose and breathes life into the pages as they turn.

Another concept of note, and which relates to the individual giving reality meaning, is the distinction between fact and fiction. As you may imagine, this book draws heavily on stories and ideas about Vikings and ninjas. Now, the popular conception of who they were and what they did is likely very different from the historical reality. But does it matter? Maybe if you were an historian aiming to accurately portray the past, yet if our goal is motivation and direction, I'm not so sure. Regardless, the information here is a mixture of reality and fantasy, drawing from history and popular culture. If you're looking for a textbook, go back to the library. We've all been inspired by fictional characters and ideas, and that's because they're often more real, more pure, than what we encounter in everyday life.

A book, however, remains a book. While this one focuses heavily on philosophy, Viking Ninja is equally oriented around fitness and the human body. Physical instruction, or at least practice—will be key to your development and flourishing within the system should you choose to participate. You can't learn to use the mace without ever holding one, nor can you obtain ninja-like movement skills if you sit on the couch all day and can't touch your toes. Whether you visit a workshop or stick to videos is up to you, but motion is imperative.

This text is just the beginning. Though reading it is an important step, it's meaningless without the journey that follows, which is the true substance of experience. Employ what you learn and discover here in your daily life. Practice it, and seek out people with whom you can share ideas. Growth is vacuous without love and community. Make that central to your training and you are guaranteed to succeed.

- Robinson Erhardt

VIKING

"Viking" is one of the two core elements of Viking Ninja. It reflects the steel mace and the energy required to wield it. When you're working with a mace, you're not just training for fitness—you're preparing for combat, the battle within. We're here to wage war against our weaknesses.

The Viking age began at the end of the eighth century when the Scandinavians began attacking lands across the sea. Their raids were unanticipated, as Europeans never believed it was possible to make such a voyage and attack their coasts. In 793, the English scholar Alcuin wrote to Aethelred, the King of Northumbria: "Lo, it is nearly three hundred and fifty years that we and our fathers have inhabited this most lovely land, and never before has such terror appeared in Britain as we have suffered from a pagan race, nor was it thought that such an inroad from sea could be made."

The Vikings defied the impossible by bending reality to their vision. We all have dreams and goals, and though they may be across the sea, the only thing that can stop us from achieving them is the strength—or weakness—of our wills. Limitations exist only in the mind, and the Vikings had the strength to crash through them with force never before seen by the world. Every time we pick up a mace, enter the gym, or simply open our eyes to the morning, we have to be possessed of the same motive force.

Viking warriors were buried with their sword, mace, or axe, as it was thought they would need it with them in Valhalla, the afterlife. If a warrior died without his weapon in hand it was considered a disgrace. According to the historian Ewart Oakeshott, "The hard-headed Norse people [believed that] a man should not inherit his father's treasures, but should go out and win his own, lest he grow soft and lazy."

When we emulate the Viking, our goal is to put honor first before everything else. We don't want to live on the backs of our fathers. We aim to go forth and make a name by pushing ourselves as far as our bodies, minds, and spirits will take us. We fight to become legendary.

Contrary to popular belief, the Vikings were not primarily warriors but farmers. Everyone had to grow their own food, and early on there were few professional soldiers. But that doesn't mean they were unskilled. To be a Viking —or in this case to train and improve your body, mind, and spirit—doesn't necessitate that you be "special" in any sense. Everyone has the right to be great. We were born to it. The Vikings never had anything handed to them. They ventured out into the world to take it. If you were given your strengths they would have no value. Real treasure's worth is defined by the blood, sweat, and tears it takes to achieve it.

Another dead-wrong conventional opinion about the Vikings is that they were brutish, nasty barbarians. Though they certainly didn't have good table manners based on today's norms, they were honor-bound to the end. The Vikings evolved from the barbarian tribes who plagued the Romans for centuries, of whom the historian Tacitus wrote thus: "On the field of battle it is a disgrace to the chief to be surpassed in valor by his companions or the companions not to come up in valor to their chief. As for leaving the battle alive after your chief has fallen, that means lifelong infamy and shame. To defend and protect him, put down one's own acts of heroism to his credit, that is what they really mean by allegiance."

Being part of Viking Ninja means joining a brotherhood. The Vikings fought to the last man and guarded their comrades' backs. We're all here in the same place—though it may not be physical—to achieve the same goals, and we work together to achieve them. If you aren't honest and true to that mission, then you have no business being part of the community and should go back to working the fields.

The following quote from the epic poem Beowulf does much to illustrate the high esteem in which Vikings held their weapons: "Not the least or the worst of his war equipment / Was the sword the herald of Hrothgar loaned / In his hour of need—Hrunting its name— / An ancient Heirloom, trusty and tried; / Its blade was of iron, with etched design / Tempered in blood of many a battle / Never in fight had it failed the hand / That drew it, daring the perils of war, / The rush of the foe. Not the first time then / That its edge must venture on valiant deeds."

We have to take the same attitude every day. Certainly, we must treat our maces, our fitness equipment, as if our lives depend on them. After all, they are the tools we use to surpass ourselves. But we must also take care of our minds, bodies, and spirits—not just the material weapons we wield. Our homes and gyms must be clean and organized. That which we experience out in the world will inevitably effect our internal experience, our emotions and passion. A cluttered life breeds a cluttered mind.

Despite all our misconceptions, there are plenty of conventional beliefs about Vikings that appear to be accurate.

Their strength was only compounded by combat experience, as Vikings swung their swords and other weapons every day of their lives from the time they could walk. They were almost universally described as brutally strong beyond anything their foes had ever experienced. Indeed, they have what we at the gym might call farmer strength, which makes sense—they were farmers, after all—and nothing beats countless hours of hard manual labor.

In Viking Ninja we aim for this same effortless strength by prioritizing volume when we train. The body can only be as strong as the mind, and the more repetitions we put in, the greater the connection between brain and body, as we recruit muscle units to move more efficiently and powerfully.

Vikings are universally viewed as fearless warriors. There were exceptions, but the rule appears to stand strong. In Sverris saga we read, "The farmer said, 'In every battle where you are present, one of two things will happen: you will either fall or come away alive. Be bold, therefore, for everything is preordained. Nothing can bring a man to his death if his time has not come, and nothing can save one doomed to die. To die in flight is the worst death of all."

Even while at war you're in control. This comes from the mind. You have to revel in rotation and celebrate the chaos. It's all about mastering yourself through discipline—the composure to keep going even when it hurts, to maintain proper form when every part of your body is screaming to let go and relax. If you can master the mental aspect of warfare, of pushing yourself past your limits, then you enter every battle knowing you've already won, and there can be no defeat.

The Viking aspect is the strongest element of Viking Ninja because it's the powerhouse element of energy. As you can tell, everything about the Vikings revolved around strength. They had strong wills, as you couldn't sail across the sea to a foreign world, prepared to fight and defeat whatever you found there, if you didn't have conviction both in yourself and your brothers, as well as in the value of your mission. They had rugged bodies, as is evidenced by their victories and the universal lamentations of the soldiers who had to meet them in battle. And they had strong spirits, because they never gave up, no matter how hard the fight or how insurmountable the odds.

Still, the Viking element doesn't mean going hard all the time, because Vikings weren't just brutal. That's a myth huge in popular culture. They were smart, they were strategic, and they were generals. Despite their poor manners they were considered to possess crisp intelligence. Though we don't often associate the Vikings with philosophy or science, the value they placed on knowledge is one we in turn must reflect in our own lives.

Their vision wasn't psychopathic. It was about restoring their homeland, finding opportunity for their people, and standing out in the world. And they did that. We seek to do the same, though more often than not on a smaller scale. Can you reclaim your body, mind, and spirit in the pursuit of reorienting yourself toward a full, satisfying life?

The answer is a resounding yes, and that's what power means to Viking Ninja. The Warrior Spirit keeps you strong and connected to every last part of your body. It's the energy that will take you to Valhalla if you commit to honoring yourself in battle. It's not about committing to death—you honor yourself by committing to victory. When you win the battle within yourself, your energy grows and with it your strength.

But there are two sides to that coin. There's a brutal dark side and a calm light side. The dark side of the Viking is powerful, though not all bad. You can make positive things happen if you use it correctly. You can use it to eliminate corrupt people from your life, those who only bring hate and negativity. The danger grows when we lose control and do malicious things ourselves just because we feel entitled to it. That's cancer: when your heart goes black and you can't return from it.

Viking manifests itself in the system most directly through training with the steel mace. You honor the weapon to help reach the level the Vikings used to conquer the cold North. As you grow stronger, the mace will become part of you like a Marine and his rifle. You commit yourself to get the best possible results. That Marine won't be effective if he isn't tied to his tool. He'll get killed.

Training with the mace teaches you who you really are. Working with it will reveal where your Viking self lies and where you're weak. Tap into your intention and identify the power within. We all need to find that.

EXCEED YOUR LIMITATIONS

A painting of Bruce Lee hangs on the wall of my living room, and on it is the following quote:

> "You might as well be dead. Seriously, if you always put limits on what you can do, physically or anything else, it'll spread over into the rest of your life. It'll spread into your work, into your morality, into your entire being. There are no limits. There are plateaus, but you must not stay there, you must go beyond them. If it kills you, it kills you. A man must constantly exceed his level."

I read these words every morning without fail. They resonate deep within me. The idea they convey is the entire purpose of Viking Ninja. It's why I get up in the morning. It's the stem of the flower and the root of the tree. Without this attitude I couldn't continue. It gives life meaning.

Just talking about it makes me emotional. I'm vulnerable here because we're dissecting the core of my being. And in the end that's okay. I'm proud to share how I feel, because that's what it's all about. Even this constitutes exceeding my limits, as my instinct is to close up and keep these thoughts inside.

If any paragraph describes the Warrior Spirit, it's this one, and the Warrior Spirit is central to Viking Ninja. No person without it amounts to anything. The Warrior Spirit isn't a complacent thing—it always strives to improve, to learn and absorb everything that will make it stronger. If this sounds familiar, that's because it's nearly identical to Onnit's mission of Total Human Optimization. To truly optimize yourself and honor your Warrior Spirit, you need three things: commitment, discipline, and dedication.

First comes commitment. You're reading this book, which is a start. Maybe you already own a mace or have even trained with me in the past. But to succeed in your goals you must be steadfast like a boulder that braves a crashing river decade after decade without shifting an inch. This doesn't mean you have to swing the mace every day, but you must be prepared to make movement a vital part of your existence. Without integrating it into your life, you will never master your body, and without pursuing mastery you cannot nurture your Warrior Spirit.

Training is no easy task. It hurts, and you will have to push yourself. This is where discipline comes in. Some days you won't want to work, but those are the days you need it most. Any lapse in discipline is a tiny fracture in the bridge between you and optimization. Enough cracks and it will collapse, preventing you from crossing. With time you may rebuild that bridge, but it's not the easy path to take.

Yet the self-control necessary to honor your Warrior Spirit extends beyond the mace, the nunchucks, and even the barbell. You will have to nourish your body with diet and exercise, feed your mind through the pursuit of knowledge and rest when required. This will ultimately be a lifelong journey and require a strong will, along with time and energy. Find your power and cultivate the proper mindset.

The last piece is dedication. You must commit yourself to your craft, to the pursuit of excellence in all you do. You've already accepted your training, but that's not enough—it's the bare minimum. You're disciplined enough to complete the tasks before you, to remain engaged with your work. But beyond that you must be dedicated. You must give your all each and every time you pick up the mace. You must live your best life through your chosen tool.

In practice, developing excellence demands patience. You will work every day to sculpt your ideal body—one that can fight, work, and love with the power of a thousand-year storm. Patience is no easy thing, yet it's crucial for anyone seeking immortality. Great things don't happen overnight, rather they require cultivation. You are growing an oak tree from an acorn, which needs rich soil and sunlight, protection from fire and poison. Every lapse is a setback.

This shouldn't be discouraging, but inspiring. Can you truly value anything that's simply handed to you? Looking back, you will see all the work you did, the pieces of yourself you left behind and put into your craft. Still, the Viking Ninja system, this lifestyle in general, is so stimulating and immersive that when you begin reaching your goals you'll turn around and think: *Where did all the time go? How did I get here?* That's the power of hard work. It may be difficult, yet the reward is the flow of losing yourself in the legacy you're building.

For all this talk, Viking Ninja is anything but that. It's about results. It's about moving and working, fighting with every breath you take. There's a time for reflection, but before reflection comes action. You must earn the right to sit back and relax, and that will come. Right now, no matter who you are, it's time to battle for improvement, to live every moment to its fullest.

With regard to getting older—that's exactly what we're fighting against. If you seek the fountain of youth, look no further. In old age come shaky hands and atrophied muscles. You can no longer grip the wheel and you lack the mental clarity to express your philosophy. We seek to battle deterioration in all its forms, instead aiming to strengthen our hold on life until it can't get away.

To conquer time, to conquer the aging process, to conquer the gravity driving you into the ground—that's the final battle, and it's just one part of the war against the self. As a Viking Ninja you must defeat your weaknesses not only to live another day, but to wage that next battle stronger and smarter than the last.

Fearlessness comes from practicing the same movements thousands of times, as with repetition comes reliable knowledge of your capacity. You know you've worked hard for your achievements, and your abilities will always be waiting at a moment's notice. This is why you might sleep with a mace at your bedside. It doesn't matter what's on the opposite side of the door—you have your weapon and the skills to use it.

On the other hand, you will have a healthy level of caution. Now you know what you're capable of—and if that's not something to fear, what is? You have the ability to cause serious damage, and this power must be treated responsibly. Yet you also know what others with similar training can do. People out there may wish to do you harm, and you must be prepared for them.

In the end you will find harmony, like water. You will have the ability to assert yourself, showing aggression when threatened, while also understanding when to be reserved. While the novice may strike at anything in reach, the well-trained warrior sits back until action is necessary. Not everything that barks must be confronted—it's only the things that bite. Finding this balance is harder than it sounds, yet fundamental to the system.

The humility that comes with grasping the extent of one's own abilities is integral not only to your relationship with the world, but also with yourself. As soon as you stop trying to prove your value to everyone who walks past, you can focus more deeply on self-betterment. It is thus that harnessing your ego is the first step to opening the gate that leads toward unimaginable strength.

You won't exceed your level every time you face a test. Failure is inevitable. It's all about progression, little by little. The goal is to constantly challenge your emotions, your body, your mind. Stay real and never give in.

This quote centers me like yin and yang. The black and white are constantly in motion trying to swallow one another, and thus they propel each other forward in perpetual balance. Bruce Lee's words push me to exceed my limitations. Every time you hit a landmark in life, whenever you feel resistance, whenever the thought creeps into your mind that maybe you can't go any further, that's when you press harder than ever before. That's when you kill the voice, the ego, and challenge your discipline to reach the next level.

This is where you dig deep mentally, spiritually, and physically, where you find out who you really are. Can you move past the talk and execute the walk? If you're only doing it for the fame, for selfishness, for compliments, it won't fuel the journey you have to take. You're on a rowboat trying to cross the sea. But if passion fuels your dedication, your discipline, your months and years of practice, then you're sailing on a solid Viking craft with fifty men working around the clock pumping the oars.

Are you dedicated enough to keep chipping away at those barriers, or do you give up and move on to the next one, the next one, the next one. Bruce Lee didn't fear the man who knew ten thousand kicks, but the man who threw the same kick ten thousand times. That's dangerous. That's how you grow sharp and turn from ninja to samurai. Exceeding your limits doesn't mean saying, "Hey, I sit on the couch sixteen hours a day bathing in cheetos, so I'm going to have a stick of celery and call it a victory." It means never resting until you've achieved your dreams and made a difference in the world. Exceeding your limits is the staple that binds this book together.

I feed off this quote every single day. I feed off this attitude, this mindset. Strength is what makes me tick. I feed off the strength to survive. Mental strength. Versatility. Durability. My goal is to find leaks of strength and destroy them. Every step back is two steps you must take to move forward. I kill weakness. I kill the ego. I challenge my discipline.

Some people may read this and think hard work won't make them happier. But it's not about being happier. Happiness is on everyone's mind, and yet nobody knows what it is or how to achieve it. Otherwise we'd all be there, wouldn't we? You have to think outside the box and try things you haven't done before. What this attitude will do is give you the discipline necessary to find fulfillment. Satisfaction, self-honesty, self-love—they're all way undervalued in comparison to happiness. If you want immediate gratification, grab a donut. It won't last. But if you want to sleep well at night, eager for the next day and the challenges that await you, then be prepared to give your all from the moment you wake up until the moment you tuck yourself in at night.

This extends beyond the big things in life. It's not just about getting your black belt, writing a book, or landing a new job. The human body is lazy. We have too much freedom. Your phone does your socializing, the microwave your cooking. If you had a robot to wipe your butt for you... well, you get the picture. We need to dial back into ourselves. We need to work hard. Forget the microwave. Start cooking. Get out and train with your friends. Embrace the inconvenient and find your grind.

THE VALKNUT

The moment I laid eyes on the Valknut I knew it was a symbol of great power, and one I would incorporate into the structure and philosophy of Viking Ninja. You can find the image on the back cover of the book. Within the system it embodies the mind.

The Valknut has its origins with the Vikings and their barbarian ancestors, and is most often associated with the god Odin. It represented his superior mental abilities and his power to manipulate and control both himself and those around him. His mind-bind, it was said, sent the Vikings to war and kept them committed to their tasks without succumbing to distraction.

The Valknut anchors the pillars of Viking Ninja philosophy. Each triangle contains a trinity of concepts that function synergistically while also contributing to the whole. Yet the ideas are unbound, constantly in flux. The three triangles have to be united in order to find balance, and thus your purpose.

The top point of the first triangle is the *weapon*. A warrior is nothing without his mace, hands, or whatever else he uses for combat. Skills must be cultivated so that when war comes the Viking can spring into action confident he can wield his weapon to its potential.

Inherent to the weapon is battle. When we use a

weapon, the most important battle isn't external—it's inside us. We're waging a war against our own heads to remain in control. Physically this manifests itself as we struggle to maintain our structure, which any type of motion will seek to compromise. If we lose our physical structure then we lose everything, which will be reflected immediately in our mental composure.

Second in this trinity is *trophy*. Historically speaking, the mace wasn't only used as a tool, but as an object of reverence signifying authority. If you don't revere your weapon, you can't learn from and grow with it. How many people at your gym carelessly toss their equipment around? They don't respect their peers, their temple, or the tool they work with. Keep your weapon in prime condition for when you need it most.

Just like a sword, give your mace a sheath. Though you will ultimately gain your might from within, the mace must be respected for the power it bestows upon you. Whether taking care of your weapon means sharpening your blade, scrubbing your callouses, or polishing your nunchucks, the extent to which you succeed in your development will not exceed the degree to which you care for your materials.

Third is the concept of *power*. First you must honor your weapon by studying it. Then you must treat it with adoration. Yet without strength and ability, your hands are useless. The barbell is dead weight. A mace is nothing but a symbol. It may take time to understand and love the tool, but eventually you will develop the coordination necessary to use it properly, and with this comes the responsibility to be safe and wield your weapon only for good.

The mace has a long and storied history. It was essentially the first weapon ever created, as it's a close cousin of the club, and has thus been used since the dawn of man. Among the most well-known maces in history is the Indian

Gada, which was swung by the Hindu god Hanuman. His followers trained day and night with the mace hoping they might one day achieve a similar degree of power.

The next trinity involves three types of rotation you will learn more about when you begin working directly with the mace, though they can apply to any tool. On an abstract level, these rotational aspects extend to the way in which the world influences you and the corresponding force you exert back upon it.

The first type of rotation is *anti-rotation*. When dealing with offset weight your body will be pulled in various directions, and you must fight to remain immobile. The same concept applies to life—you must master your mind, body, and spirit to become an immovable force. Otherwise you are nothing more than a leaf in the wind, bending to any and everything around you.

After anti-rotation comes *counter-rotation*. While the former means isolating your body, the latter requires resisting whatever seeks to press you. When the mace pulls left, you employ equal and opposite force to push right. This way you maintain agency no matter what you encounter. Similarly to our leaf in the wind, you fight back against influences outside your control, nullifying them by counterbalancing their intent.

The final element in this trinity is *purposeful rotation*. Once you've stabilized your body and fought off anything that seeks to thwart your sovereignty, you can initiate rotation yourself. This pertains to exercises like the uppercut—striking, attacking movements—where you leave your base of support to engage your opponent. Though to survive and flourish it is necessary to protect yourself, you cannot live by those skills alone, as then you are little more than a stone—unbending and rigid. You must also exert your will on the world.

Though the trinities work together, ebbing and flowing as one, the third triangle is the most significant of the Valknut. Its first point is the *body*, without which you can't swing your weapon or protect yourself in any capacity. It is of paramount importance to keep yourself in the best possible shape. This means respecting your nutrition, training, sleep, recovery, and anything else that contributes to the state of your physical form.

The second part of the last trinity is the *mind*. As I like to say, most bodies don't have a mind, and most minds don't have a body. At many gyms you find vain individuals focused only on their appearance and little else, sacrificing the intellectual aspect of the equation, while in most library dungeons you find the opposite—those who neglect the physical world in the pursuit of abstractions. Without a sound mind, how can you know when, how, or why to use your body? The two are intrinsically connected, and both integral to the warrior.

The final piece of this triangle is *intent*, which bridges the mind and body, and can also be thought of as the spirit. All you need to move is a body, and with a mind you have the knowledge to do so, but the spirit is what gives flavor to this ability. You've mastered purposeful rotation, but can you use it? Deprived of intent you're little more than a machine, capable of great things but bereft of the fire required to accomplish them. All nine aspects of the Valknut are required to unify the Viking.

Without the mind-bind our heads are full of chaos, and that's exactly what comes out if we can't control ourselves. It's a one-way path, and not the kind you want to be on. If you don't master your mind-bind, then you will never find success. Thus, the first key is understanding the Valknut. Without knowledge of the problem, how can you hope to solve it? The three interlocking triangles represent nine distinct elements that are in a constant state of flux. They have to be locked down, isolated, and tied to one another in order to be functional rather than chaotic.

Although they don't form their own triangle, dedication, commitment, and discipline are necessary to give the Valknut form and keep it from becoming a mess. This is a familiar theme in the philosophy. Dedication comes from your heart, and gives you the strength to put all your effort toward something meaningful.

With dedication comes commitment. It's not enough to simply apply yourself—you have to give it your all every moment. If any weakness shows itself in your mind-bind, everything will crumble to pieces. It only takes one chink in the dam before the waters come flooding through to drown the village below.

Discipline enables that commitment and keeps the mind-bind in order. This, above any other quality, is key to success. Discipline is the antithesis of aimlessness, and provides the scaffolding with which you can right your mind and organize its pieces.

We all know how difficult it is to keep trudging forward when we don't see an end in sight. But discipline, dedication, and commitment are predicated on there being an end. Without a path, without a purpose, how can you hope to maintain the Valknut in order? Without structure, water crashes and flows formlessly, but the moment you give it a cup to fill it finds its form.

This is a perfect example of how the elements in this philosophy are tightly bound together. If one piece in the Valknut overpowers another, it all falls apart. Each of the triangles has its purpose. This is where balance enters the equation, ensuring the Valknut's elements are in harmony so that the mind-bind doesn't degrade. But this is a topic for a later section.

I don't actively think about the Valknut when I'm training. If you're in the moment, stay there. Don't leave it to ponder anything else, as distractions are how you get injured and fail to achieve your goals. That doesn't mean the Valknut is unimportant for your physical journey, however. I always consider the Valknut before I begin my day's training. It's not necessarily a conscious thing, as I don't go through every point in my mind. Rather I consider the whole and what it represents.

When most of us warm up, and certainly when we work out, our minds are all over the place. What am I going to eat after class? I should go talk to that girl. Do my biceps look big? This is a recipe for disaster. Or, if disaster is too extreme, it's certainly a recipe for wasted time. As I warm up, I think about my body, as my primary goal is self-improvement and maintaining safety. Still, that's only part of it. I don't exclusively watch the breath. I don't play music. I consider my mind-bind. I gauge whether or not I'm centered and focused, or how I can achieve that state if I'm not. When my brain is all over the place I have to reset my intention to ensure that my training has purpose and I'm working toward something. I can't let chaos take over if I want to grow while also setting an example for others.

The Valknut is a tool for calming your mind and re-engaging your focus. It's a major part of my lifestyle. As a therapeutic symbol, it reminds me of how prone we are to unbridled thoughts. Understanding the concept enables you to strengthen yourself mentally to cope with the stresses of life and prepare for them in the future.

Everything about the Valknut aims toward and contributes to flawless execution. Without having all these qualities in line, neither the Vikings nor the ninjas would have been as successful as they were. They couldn't have remained orderly. Without a settled mind there is only chaos, and with chaos comes destruction, not execution.

VIKING NINJA

The name for my system was given to me at Onnit, where Aubrey Marcus called me the Viking Ninja. I'm half Norwegian and half Mongolian, so it makes sense. I hear I look the part, too. The way I see it, two lines of warriors run in my blood—the Vikings and the Mongols.

Yet those two cultures brought chaos to the world. I want to take another route and bring humanity something great with the best medicine there is—physical activity. Being physically active reprograms your body, unlocking longevity. You can live to be a hundred and still feel amazing, but for that you have to be responsible. Viking Ninja aims to provide that—a revolutionary process to improve your functionality.

The Mongols sought to rule the world, and the Vikings aimed to conquer it. If the ideas behind this system were to find their way into every heart, if they resonated within every soul they touched, it would become a platform for dedication, the promise to progress, the commitment to growth. Viking Ninja means taking every last bit of yourself and applying it toward living your best life. That means working hard to become stronger and last longer.

At its core, the system centers around fitness. That, however, doesn't mean the body is our only priority. On the contrary, the mind and spirit are every bit as important to this enterprise we're embarking on. Yet it's a lot easier to change the way your muscles move and function than how you think and feel, and therein lies the key. By training the body, by learning to kill the ego and challenge your discipline, we access the difficult-to-reach realm of mind and spirit through the readily available and tangible physical world.

The goal of fitness is strength: being adaptable and flexible when necessary, but strong and unbending as well. Viking Ninja is about defeating the forces that aim to crush you. It's about defeating rot. It's about being able to resist oppression by taking your life back in your hands and being responsible for your actions rather than letting the cards fall as they will. It's about being both the redwood that withstands centuries of fire and storm and the tiger that delves into the thickest jungle and takes what it needs to thrive.

You have to own your life, to be fearless and appreciate your capabilities as a human being. We only have one shot, and we can't jump into anyone else's shoes. Social media and popular culture have become an epidemic, a disease of epic proportions. Rather than living our own lives, we spend more and more of our time trying to escape into others'. We worship at the feet of the strong, the attractive, the successful rather than doing what it takes to achieve that same level.

When we apply ourselves, whether it's through work or fitness, we rarely do it for ourselves. We want money for shoes to impress our friends. We want muscles so that we can flex on Instagram. That's not the Viking Ninja way. I want to make life real again. I want you to create for the sake of it, to train so that you can be strong for yourself and the people you love, not for something so meaningless as a like or a share.

You have to use your body to the utmost while taking care of it to the same extent. This goes for the mind and spirit as well. Integral to the system is taking responsibility for yourself in all areas of life. If you drive a Ferrari, you have to pay a higher insurance premium. That goes for maintenance, too. The more successful or competitive the athlete, the more time they have to spend healing their bodies.

So many of us drive ourselves into the ground because we neither take care of ourselves after exercise nor aim to recover from the chronic stresses of modern life. If you think sitting for eight hours a day hunched in front of a screen doesn't take its toll on your spinal health, when you're sixty years old and can't take a step without pain explain to me how you got there. Unlike so many systems, we aim to look at both sides of the coin—performance, certainly, but also recovery.

Even though there's so much emphasis on the individual, Viking Ninja revolves around community. World domination comes when everybody not only worries about improving themselves, but those around them, which is where brotherhood becomes so important. We can only go so far on our own. We all stand on the backs of the giants who came before us.

Viking Ninja couldn't have been born without a whole pantheon of gods and thinkers in the world of fitness and martial arts. Without Bruce Lee, the Vikings and ninjas themselves, the millions who died in combat over the course of history, we wouldn't be where we are today. But the same thing goes on a much more microcosmic level. Without teachers to learn from or friends to motivate and push you, the extent to which you can grow will be severely curbed. And where is the joy in finding success if you have no one to celebrate with?

Viking Ninja does not discriminate. There's a place for everyone who wants to better themselves and has a thirst for knowledge and self-discovery. Physically, our goals are to correct imbalances and movement deficiencies. It's also about finding proper structure and activation. You can only expect to live so long and so healthily if your spine curves like a snake. And if you lack the basic strength and coordination to squat properly, to move heavy objects, then you're setting yourself up for fast-paced deterioration as you age. These basic comforts are accessible to anyone if they're willing to commit themselves. And after that, only the sky's the limit.

Most people are starting from square one. They're injured, insecure, and clueless. We have to respect that and say, "Hey, it's not your fault. We're here for you. We want to help." Nobody can choose the life they were born into, the family that raised them, the influences that shaped them. But there comes a point in everyone's life where they have to step forth and put their foot down. They have to say, "I've had enough and I'm ready to take responsibility for myself." Viking Ninja is about answering that call.

What makes an education, fitness, or other system good? I believe if it accepts everyone's individuality while still being able to help anybody who comes in reach their goals, it's a great system. All systems must be bound by rules, and with that comes a theme for helping the general population. The leeway and wiggle room comes with regression and progression.

Everybody needs to know how to squat, for example, but we all start somewhere different, and we all have idiosyncrasies that need correction. If you just had a hip replacement and aren't ready to do a hundred repetitions with a twenty-five pound mace in each hand, there's no shame in that. Regression isn't failure—it's a step toward the success any given person is working toward. It's a success for you as a coach if you enable someone to grow without injuring or otherwise harming them. But certain people take that as a failure because they don't think they reached the end goal. This is a perfect situation in which the phrase, "Kill your ego, challenge your discipline," needs to be heard loud and clear.

If you don't reward yourself for completing a regression, you'll never commit to the progression. If you have a coach, that's great, but if you don't you have to be both the donkey and the person holding the carrot on a stick at the same time.

Killing the ego means self-acceptance. You have to understand where you are and where you're going. If you won't accept that you just had your hip replaced and you want to be doing the same program as Donald Cerrone, then this isn't the place for you. I'm not going to take responsibility when you get hurt. That being said, we're here to help you find yourself, and from there exceed your limits. But we all have to start somewhere, and deluding yourself will only get you injured and frustrated, not results.

Our basic fitness goals for everyone are the same—performance and durability—though they will look different depending on the person. If you're an eighty year old couch potato, you may not have the same needs as a star NFL player, but that's why Viking Ninja is what it is. We want everyone to excel in the same fundamental categories. Where they go from there is up to them. You need to develop strength throughout a wide range of motion. Everyone must be able to defend themselves. Everyone needs to foster an awareness of their body and its capabilities.

Viking Ninja differs from other systems not only because of our attention to regression and progression, but because of our emphasis on volume. And this volume is not just in terms of repetitions and sets, but the volume of demand, discipline, and dedication we expect from our coaches and athletes. It all centers around health-first fitness through high-volume, low-impact training. That means safety, which is a prerequisite for all movement.

We're training to improve our lives, not get hurt in the gym, which defeats the purpose in the first place. You will learn that a fast heart rate is nothing more than that. It can have a purpose, yet too often we equate breaking a sweat with self-improvement.

Though Viking Ninja is expressive and demanding, we are responsible in training. You can have fun, but you have to be careful and attentive. Remaining disciplined in your practice is key not only to finding progress, but also to preserving your body. If you zone out, you're not digging deep enough or in the right place. Instead of mining for gold you're off in the desert searching for sand. Our programming centers around mindfulness.

Though it's hard work, the adrenaline you get from proper training is addicting. Getting strong is just as much about seeking strength as it is striving to eliminate weakness. Before fitness, the philosophy has to make sense. The mind first, then the body. If there's any disconnection your training will be unrewarding and unsatisfying.

With growth comes suffering, and with suffering comes a dark road. You have to be prepared for that. The journey will not be easy. But when people go down that dark road they'll have brothers and sisters to provide them with a flashlight. That way they can locate the path before them, and with community they're able to get on it once more. Then they can reinvent themselves into something extraordinary.

WARRIOR SPIRIT

Nurturing the Warrior Spirit is fundamental to Viking Ninja. It's such an intuitive concept that I'm always surprised when people ask about it. To me it's obvious. Engaging the Warrior Spirit means digging deep into your body to find the next level of your existence. How strong can you be? How much energy can you put forth? How fast can you go and how hard can you work? It means always pushing yourself, no matter where you're at, and bringing out something more.

The Warrior Spirit is your root. It's the source of your integration. You access it in the middle of a fight, at the heart of war, in the thrusts of battle, as you grapple to become better than you were the moment before. We find it whenever we're in the midst of a struggle. If you're dieting and have cravings, you activate the part of you that knows what you need to do. Then you push through that desire because it's only at the surface level. If there's work to be done, you push through the weakness that tells you to sit on your bum and instead you activate the inner killer that feeds off of purpose.

As Viking Ninja is inherently a fitness system, we strive to bring out the Warrior Spirit through movement. It's the energy that allows you to sprint the last mile of a marathon after you've already given everything you have to make it through the first twenty-five. And the Warrior Spirit is what would allow you to run the entire course again back to the finish line if something or someone you loved were in danger.

Nothing can defeat the Warrior Spirit if you tap into it properly. It's a massive, chaotic force. It's what lets mothers rip off car doors when their children are trapped inside. We all have it, and we all know that we can access it to drive the best from us and find the next level of possibility. If you think you're finished, that you've given everything, then you're only halfway there. Remember that the human soul is the most powerful thing on earth. The body may be fragile, but the will can push it farther than we ever think possible.

Yet no matter how powerful the mind may be, it inhabits a physical body that has needs. As Peter Parker's Uncle Ben said, "With great power comes great responsibility." You're the the director, the driver, the leader. Sometimes you have to slow down. Sometimes you have to speed up. Sometimes volume rises, and other times it's intensity.

Just because your mind can push you to complete a triathlon every day for a month doesn't mean you should do it. The Warrior Spirit understands balance, and pushing past that is the result of the ego trying to prove something. On the other end you have the fear of failure, which keeps you from living up to your potential. Your Warrior Spirit knows the importance of honesty by ensuring that you shove aside fear to reach your potential, but it also remembers balance to prevent you from going harder than is safe just to satisfy your pride at the expense of your wellbeing.

The Warrior Spirit is your deepest self. Fear will keep you from reaching it. Pain, fatigue, excuses—your lack of discipline—will keep you from reaching it. All these things kill the Warrior Spirit. You need to overcome those obstacles to bring out your best self. It doesn't happen in one day, and that's why we train. That's why we unite and help each other. That's why we're truthful to a fault and call out our brothers and sisters on their shortcomings. We're all here to grow, and I want people in my life who will be honest with me, not who will coddle me just to make themselves feel better.

If I commit to hard training I follow my plan. Yet that also means I have to be reasonable when I design it. If you're obese can you starve yourself for six months to lose your excess weight? Yes, but is that healthy for your mind, soul, or body? No, and making that your plan is irresponsible and unfair to the Warrior Spirit.

When used properly, the Warrior Spirit brings you the intention and integration necessary for success. But no matter how well you plan, there will be hitches along the way. You have to be aware, present, attentive. If a training program makes me breathe too hard and I'm on the verge of death, why would I keep moving as fast as my legs can take me? I need to dial it down and keep my brain intact.

Though we all have the Warrior Spirit, it's something that needs to be trained. If you've never run a mile in your life, how can you expect to adequately plan your route when you have no idea what your capacity is? The more we tap into our Warrior Spirit to push through limitations, the better we understand ourselves and the better we're able to use that drive going forward.

We train the Warrior Spirit with progression and regression. First you have to find out where your limits are. Then you figure out how to overcome them. Afterward it's all about effort. Are you really searching for the greater you, that final piece necessary to accomplish your goals? Are you fighting to finish, or are you finished already? These are the qualities I look for in someone's attitude.

How do we eliminate weaknesses and find a stronger path toward a new mindset? Open up bandwidth for creativity and strength by destroying fear. We're all held back by past trauma, by the ego, by wanting to save face and preserve appearances. Yet if you never apply yourself, you'll never find the walls of your cage. And if you never push against those walls, you'll never break them.

The next step is connecting the mind and body. They can't be separate. You have to go all in. There are no cop-outs, no half-baked attempts at progress. Commitment takes dedication, and with dedication come rewards. Once your mind and body are linked, you can utilize that limitless well of power in the human soul to push yourself to find the health and vigor of body that you always wanted, to live long and powerfully.

Vikings embody the Warrior Spirit. They went into battle without fear. That meant they already won. Their hearts were in it a hundred percent regardless of whether or not they would actually be victorious because they'd already won in their minds. That's why they were so dangerous. They couldn't lose. If their commander died, they'd fight to the last man just for the sake of honor. We have to foster that same attitude. When we go into battle, whatever that means for us, we have to go in knowing we will give everything we have, and that thus no matter what the outcome is we've won the battle against the self, against internal weakness and the ego.

The ninjas' Warrior Spirit came in the form of their commitment to execution. They were precise, and that took unbelievable discipline. They did not make mistakes, because mistakes meant death. Ninja represents the discipline of the Warrior Spirit, whereas Viking represents the strength, the battle, the fearlessness. When you put those two together you're unstoppable. Ninja is tactical, Viking is brutal. Ninja is organized, Viking is chaotic. There's nothing more powerful than controlled chaos.

I tap into the Warrior Spirit the moment I wake up. You have to accept it as soon as your day begins. Maybe your hip hurts. Maybe it's your back. You could be tired. Something might be on your mind. Are your feelings hurt? Job suck? You're going to be confronted with challenges from the moment you step out of bed. You have to decide right then and there to defeat them. Win the battle before it starts.

Some mornings you'll wake up happy, but that doesn't mean the whole day will go smoothly. Be prepared. Walk out the door knowing exactly who you are, what you're going to do, and how you'll handle yourself. Go for it a hundred percent. If you go eighty you're going to fail, and people will take advantage of you. The Warrior Spirit doesn't know eighty percent. It only knows a hundred percent, though what it also knows is balance, meaning that it will give whatever it needs, no more and no less, to navigate any potential situation.

My friend Carlos Condit of the UFC was born with the Warrior Spirit, and you know that if you've ever seen him fight in the Octagon. Carlos's war never ends. He's a grinder. He stays in the pocket of hell. He knows how to control his chaos. He knows how to be calm through the storm. He knows how to strike impeccably. They call him the Natural Born Killer, yet in real life he's the most wonderful, generous gentleman you could ever meet. That's balance.

The Warrior Spirit comes out the moment you decide not to be a victim anymore. No one was born to be a pushover. The Warrior Spirit is like a single mother. They have to deal with three kids and one job. Every day she has to find the warrior within to keep that operation going.

There are few people in the world I admire more than single mothers, because it's not easy to keep going like that twenty-four seven, especially when everything you do is for other people.

TOTAL HUMAN OPTIMIZATION

Viking Ninja was born under the umbrella of Onnit. Their mission, as stated by Aubrey Marcus, is "to inspire peak performance through a combination of unique products and actionable information. Combining bleeding-edge science, earth-grown nutrients, and time-tested strategies from top athletes and medical professionals, we are dedicated to providing our customers with supplements, foods, and fitness equipment aimed at helping people achieve a new level of well-being we call Total Human Optimization."

Just like Onnit, at Viking Ninja we strive to help the world achieve Total Human Optimization. However, we have a slightly different method of implementation. Still, our two organizations complement one another, and in this section I'd like to introduce you to the philosophy at Onnit, as well as how I interpret it, so that you can see the environment in which Viking Ninja was conceived as well as the connection to our current values.

As I see it, Total Human Optimization is like a tree. Trees, more than any other living thing, represent strength over the years. The older a tree gets, the stronger and larger it grows. It adds layers of depth and character. It's totality increases with every day that it persists.

People are like seeds trying to become complete. Optimization is the process we undergo for that to occur. We change from formless, moldable clay into unique, complex individuals as we express ourselves to the greatest degree.

Consider the tree as a human body. The entirety of the tree encompasses far more than just the bark and leaves you see. If you want to understand the tree, you have to look at its roots. If you were to uproot the tree, you would find that just as much of it is below ground as above, and that what's beneath the surface is a mirror image of the visible.

How do you optimize that tree, making it powerful enough to live for generations and surmount all the difficult conditions thrown at it by nature? For us, you have to use the mind and body, the outer world and underworld, the roots and the branches. Just as the tree is planted in the earth, we are inherently connected to our environment. The tree draws nutrients from the soil in the form of water, minerals, and other compounds. We're exposed to life, and from it we draw imagination, inspiration, sustenance.

The tree takes what it gets from the earth and turns that into pure life. It takes on color. It buds in the spring when in winter it was barren. Yet trees are far more simple than humans. They're born with plans contained inside them. There's no thinking involved. A tree simply is, and a tree simply does.

People, on the other hand, are not the same. We have to discover for ourselves how to become strong. Some trees grow tall and others die out. Some people shine bright, and other languish on the couch. When a seed is unlucky enough to set its roots in the wrong soil, it's destined to die. Its path is death, and there is no choice. People, on the other hand, don't have that dilemma. No matter where we're born, we have the power to uproot ourselves and choose our path. No matter where you are today, no matter who or what you surround yourself with, you can uproot and find more fertile soil.

We all want to be the tallest, broadest tree in the forest. And it's possible, but you have to strive. Unlike the tree, you have agency. The only destiny you have is the one you make for yourself. Total Human Optimization is about seeking out that destiny and making it a reality by drawing upon all the resources at your disposal. That requires killing your ego and challenging your discipline. Everything is circular.

The roots of Total Human Optimization are found in the pillars of the Onnit Academy, which Viking Ninja adheres to as well. The first of the five principles is Unity in Diversity. We are at our best, and strongest because of, what we draw from others. I wasn't born a Viking or a ninja, and yet I've taken from them to make myself stronger. I didn't create the mace or barbell. I learned from and studied with the greatest teachers and movers in the world. That open-mindedness is what's led Viking Ninja to become what it is today.

Both Viking Ninja and the Onnit Academy are actually anti-systems: we actively fight against dogma and arbitrary rule-making. So many schools of fitness (let alone science, art, religion, or any other field) come to believe that they are at the apex of knowledge and study, thus ignoring others' achievements. We seek to do the opposite by working with those who can inspire and teach us. The Onnit Academy itself isn't the work of just a few people—John Wolf and Shane Heins, its chief architects, drew from all manner of research and practice to structure their curriculum.

Opposite *Unity in Diversity*, Onnit aims toward *Giving to Empower*. So do we. This means sharing what we've built with others. It's all one cycle, and my work—our work—has no value if it doesn't contribute to the greater cause and improve the lives of many. I want to empower others to take what I've learned as they create their own systems and philosophies.

Onnit also strives for *Balance in Harmony*, and balance is key to Viking Ninja. This is seen in the pursuit of both performance and recovery, where the scale must be struck even for optimal results. It's also true in Onnit's fourth principle, the *Search for Truth*, where objective and subjective measurements must be evaluated to holistically assess the situation. And ultimately balance is found in the recognition that the mind, body, and spirit must be equally present in any activity for success.

Last of the Onnit Academy's pillars is *Action is Leadership*. I take this one to heart with everything I do. As the head of Viking Ninja, my words and deeds speak for more than just me. They speak for the community, and they set an example for people who share my beliefs and want to be part of something larger than themselves. We all have people who look up to us, and we thus all share this responsibility.

Though I utilize these principles to guide Viking Ninja, optimization requires leaving rules behind. To find progress you must get completely outside the box. If you do the same things you've always done, you'll end up in the exact same place. That's the whole point of unconventional training, which is what Onnit champions in the industry.

Unconventional training entails learning different ways to move our bodies, different ways to think, different ways to act outside the gym. We must be willing to change everything about our lives if we want to reach optimization. A seed doesn't become a tree by staying a seed. It sounds stupid, but people expect to achieve their goals simply by wishing them into being. That's fantasy. Actualizing dreams requires that you apply yourself and manifest reality by sheer force of will.

Moving, thinking, and being unconventionally is the key. Stress is what leads to adaptation. Squat heavy and you'll get stronger. Boil your brain in a calculus textbook and you'll get smarter. Spend time helping those less fortunate than you and your character will mature. You have to feed your body unfamiliar patterns to adapt and optimize. The same principles that apply to strength training apply everywhere else.

Total Human Optimization is a direction. The Warrior Spirit propels you to go past what you believe is possible for yourself. It starts out with something you don't think you can become, yet then you pass through it and start to believe. It's like Neo breaking through the Matrix one step at a time until he realizes he's the One. Only then he finds that his abilities extend far beyond the Matrix. It's neverending. It's about becoming that next level of human being. It's that small little bit that always keeps you from reaching Total Human Optimization. We can never reach it, because there's always one more step to go. It's the Warrior Spirit that drives us onward. The journey never ends, and that's what life is about.

You have to challenge yourself. There are no exceptions in the quest for Total Human Optimization. If you're not challenging yourself, you're not achieving excellence. You're just expressing. Expression without discipline is worthless. Anybody can make noise—who cares? What makes you different from an ape? The discipline and agency that you bring to that noise. Warrior Spirit is the intention, the commitment, the focus that propels you toward Total Human Optimization.

Onnit and Viking Ninja alike aim to support others.

We're all about family, honor, and mutual inspiration in all areas of life. It's not just health. We commit to each other. We help each other's businesses, relationships, everything you can think of. We're there for each other, and that's brotherhood. We commit to people who are willing to commit to us. That's the kind of person we hope to attract to our respective communities. We also like to help people who don't have anything, people who need us. Maybe they don't know it yet. But we'll be there for them. That's what Onnit does, and it's what we do.

Viking Ninja seeks to provide a path for everyone to reach their own definition of Total Human Optimization. As soon as you begin to engage in the system you'll discover what I mean as the optimization begins to take place. You'll feel evolution taking its course: a process that usually takes countless millennia condensed down into days, weeks, months.

Total Human Optimization applies to everything you touch, every thought you have, and every breath you take. Whether it's bodyweight movement, steel mace training, striking, cooking your breakfast, or reading a book, your intention has to be there every second of the way. You have to be engaged in your pursuit, engaged in yourself, and connecting the two if you hope to make progress and derive something meaningful from the experience.

Fundamental to Onnit's—as well as our—system is the conceptualization of all exercise in relation to longevity and performance. The former, however, is often discounted compared to the latter. Whenever we hear someone say they're training, the first thing our mind jumps to is performance. How fast can you run? How heavy can you squat? We all dream of succeeding at the highest level, though we actualize it to varying degrees. At Onnit performance must always be balanced with longevity. Excessive focus on outcomes without considering the body's needs will result in lacking progress, waning motivation, frustration, and ultimately injury.

Regardless of your goals and abilities, it is important to acknowledge this spectrum. Most of us fall somewhere in the middle. As John Wolf likes to say, unless your performance is bringing home your paycheck you should be biased toward longevity. Think of your body as a piggy bank. When you exert yourself you shake money out, and every withdrawal requires a deposit. Otherwise you're liable to go bankrupt, which is when your longevity is sacrificed and injury occurs.

Like Viking Ninja, Onnit is an expansive universe limited not only to fitness, but is open to all aspects of the mind, body, and spirit. Fitness is certainly a priority, yet we believe no one is ready for that journey until they've achieved the proper mindset to prepare them for safe, reliable, long-term progress both as an athlete and a human being.

KILL YOUR EGO

Before you can live through your Warrior Spirit, your ego must be assassinated. Ego means a lot of things, but in this instance it's the inflated sense of self-worth and importance we all possess at one time or another and that can grow to epic proportions when left unchecked.

To kill your ego means slowing down and beginning to think with your heart. We can't understand the ego until we dig consciously into all that we do. If you want to kill your ego, you have to find it first, and we're all blind when it comes to our shortcomings. It's like trying to look at your back in the mirror. The ego is a deep, necessary part of you, but it's difficult to find. You have to twist and strain.

So many of us go through our lives avoiding the hard things. That's why we bury our problems in food, drugs, or alcohol. Anything can become an addiction, a method of escape. We turn over those heavy stones in Viking Ninja by connecting to our bodies. When you push yourself to the point of breaking, everything you repress comes pouring out.

The ego lives in your subconscious, and you find it by tearing down your pride. This is easier said than done, and I don't mean to come from a high and mighty place. I'm constantly evolving, myself. I'm not the same person I was a year ago, or even a month ago. The moment you stop searching for weakness to cut away is the moment you die. It's like a bush that doesn't get pruned—eventually it will turn into a thorny mess and choke itself to death.

Don't be stubborn like that bush. Be open-minded. You have to enter into the process with the acceptance that you've failed in the past, that you're failing right now, and that these failures are going to be there waiting for you, staring you in the face, no matter where you turn. Nobody makes it through life without mistakes. You have the choice to ignore them—and thus continue making them—and suffer because of it, or you can stop dead in your tracks, take a good hard look at the mess you've left in your wake, and resolve to be more responsible going forward.

Once you find your failures, acknowledge them. There's no brushing the dust under the rug. That's the opposite of self-discovery. You can't hide from your problems. Self-honesty anchors progress, and it's necessary if you want to kill the ego.

No matter what you find inside, look it in the eye and squash it like a bug. Were you in the wrong for shouting at your spouse last night? Ignore it and you're destined to repeat yourself. The process may be hard, but you have to apologize. Did you skip your workout this morning because your bed felt too comfortable? Recognize that you aren't treating yourself well enough, get more sleep tonight, and find your way to the gym tomorrow morning. You can't change the past, but we always have power over the future.

My personal belief is that the best way to find your ego is through movement. Before you start, think about everything you do on a regular basis when you work out. What's on your mind? The most attractive person in the gym? Do you lose focus and quit whatever you're doing to perform curls by the cutest girl? If the guy next to you is squatting twice your max, do you sacrifice your health by stacking up plates to compete with him?

That's absolutely, a hundred percent, positively the wrong way to go about training and life in general. Kill that attitude. Whether you're in the gym, grocery shopping, or going on a hike, you have to fight for the best of yourself. Being distracted by other people and their accomplishments or qualities doesn't help. Don't beg for attention. That's the ego crying out like a toddler. It's not just a symptom of your obsession with others, but an inability to connect with your thoughts.

The problem with people—and I'm no exception—is that nowadays we're all begging for attention. Social media doesn't help. We're attention traders. Like my post and I'll like yours! No. None of that means a thing. If you live for others, you lose all control over yourself. We want to exceed our limitations, to strive for greatness every day. Striving for other peoples' affirmation is the opposite of that. You need to search for acceptance within your own eyes, not others'. Find that acceptance in the gym. Don't follow the sheep, or otherwise you'll end up running off a cliff. That's what happens when you place all your value in others—you can't control the outcome any longer.

If you look inside and can't find a thing to change, an aspect of pride or vanity, something ugly that needs to be killed, then you're fooling yourself because nobody's perfect. If you can't admit to your wrongs, then your ego is so big it's like the elephant in the room.

The solution? Be open-minded. This doesn't mean looking in the mirror and saying, "I have a stray hair on my eyebrow. I'll be brave and not pluck it," and then moving on with your day as if you've just made a huge accomplishment. That's better than nothing if you're the type of person who lives and dies by appearances. But this has to be a constant thing, and the deeper you look, the better. You have to get deep. Are you nasty to women because they've always turned down your advances? Do you stuff yourself with junk food because you're afraid of facing rejection? That's the real dirt you have to find, the stuff that killing will dramatically impact your life.

The ego goes through great lengths to hide insecurity. You can pay a heavy price for that, but few places will it be more dear than in the gym when your body's on the line. If you won't admit that your knee is tweaked from jiu-jitsu, after a heavy round of sprints who's to blame when you get injured? Again, that's why the gym is such a wonderful teacher for every other aspect of life. The consequences are so immediate that we can't help but learn whether we're effectively changing our character.

When ego comes first in your decision-making process it's a total giveaway that you're mentally weak. Nobody needs that. Undeserved ego is a completely different thing from earned pride. Ego wears you away with time. If you have a huge ego, your downfall will be all the greater. You'll break harder, and then you'll become a hater. We all know people who failed to achieve their dreams because they just weren't good enough, but who only went on to degrade the people who did make it. An ego that big can be smelled from a mile away, and there's nothing less attractive than unbridled arrogance. Modesty, on the other hand, is infectious. It earns admiration without even trying.

One of the most amazing athletes I've had the pleasure of working with is Earl Thomas of the NFL. He's also a terrific example of modesty in action. He's a giving man and he works hard. People say hard work is overrated, yet they couldn't be more wrong. When Earl heads to the gym it's go-time. There's no distraction. It's all dedication to practice. His discipline level is so high that he tunes out everyone else. When he has to work, he doesn't let anything get in the way. He executes like a ninja, no matter how difficult the task. The man does not make mistakes.

Still, his attitude couldn't be more humble. Lately we've been doing a lot of striking. Though Earl is a world-class athlete and football player, he's not a good boxer. But what can you expect? He's never done it before. Still, he recognizes its importance and where it stands in the Viking Ninja system. It challenges his mind and body to integrate, which is exactly what both of us want for him.

Making the mind and body work together takes serious coordination, and the better you can connect the two the better you'll perform across a wide range of tasks. And that man's connection is unbreakable. He's getting addicted to the striking, and the more addicted you are to something like that, the better your results. It doesn't just affect striking, but his game on the football field. It challenges his cardio and strengthens the relationship between eyes and hands. He now has new pathways in his nervous system. Cross-training bolsters the skills he gains from practice with his team.

And none of that would be possible if he were bowed down by pride. It may not take the shape of striking for you, or even be in the realm of fitness, but if you're closed to new possibilities you're sealing yourself off from a whole world of empowering opportunities.

THE STEEL MACE

The steel mace represents the qualities of Viking. From a fitness perspective, they had to master the technical, strength, and conditioning aspects of their chosen tool. Unfortunately the majority of what remains in the archaeological record are swords, which were the most esteemed weapons, and thus the likeliest to receive a proper burial. Children as young as three or four were buried with child-sized weapons bearing use-marks, which suggests they began training at a very young age. When war was a way of life, it wouldn't have served to be ill-prepared.

If you've never held a mace, you likely have no idea how strange the tool feels. A ten-pound mace is far heavier in the hands than a ten-pound dumbbell or kettlebell because of how the weight lies primarily at one end. Wielding it with any sort of skill requires a tremendous amount of dexterity and body awareness.

Today we often speak of farmer or old man strength, referring to people who have a preternaturally intense power level given their age and appearance. After years spent bailing hay or fixing appliances they develop a strong neuromuscular connection that drastically increases strength. From beginning to fight at such a young age, Vikings could lift and wield massive weapons that would be hard for us to swing today. We can build that degree of power with the proper progression.

The Vikings weren't a culture known for their record-keeping, yet sagas and treatises from around that time tell us they were rigorous trainers who took their warfare seriously. They practiced their motions and formations constantly to hardwire their mechanics. If the mechanics weren't right, there was only one possible outcome—their head rolled. You'd find a sword in your back, an axe in your side, or a hammer coming down between your eyes.

This is where their experience parallels what we do in the gym today. It's still strength conditioning, but by a different name. The same principles of overload, volume, and technical work apply. Contrary to popular belief, strength is absolutely a skill. There's a huge neurological component to squatting. Just because you have big muscles doesn't mean you're capable of anything. Give the man with the world's best bench press an eighty pound mace and I guarantee you he'll barely be able to swing it around his head.

Though the tool is at its core a weapon, we're using it for fitness. Still, we employ the same movements that would have been used in warfare because they are the most efficient for the body. Several biologists have postulated that humans evolved in concert with the club and spear, and that our shoulders developed for just this type of motion.

Volume's importance in training for battle is obvious. If you have a really strong swing, that's great, but what if you can only swing the mace once before you have to put it down? You're a goner. Your first couple strikes may be good, but then the third gets tired, the fourth you fatigue, and the fifth it flies from your hands. That's when you get nailed on a battlefield. Your core, your shoulders, your hands—they all have to be like iron if you want to master the tool. In the old days that meant survival. Today it means being strong, being bulletproof, being hard to kill.

Training with the steel mace revolves around skill. Dexterity is the most important of them. If you can't hold on, you're done for. You have to be able to shift the tool in your hands quickly and with precision for different patterns and ways of blocking. The battlefield is unpredictable, and you must be the same. There are tons of different grip orientations and hand-switches. If you're the type of person who likes to geek out over movement—and I certainly am—then no tool I've yet to encounter is as invigorating and stimulating as the mace.

For people interested in advanced weapons training, the steel mace is no better introduction. It's the perfect tool to engage your supporting musculature and develop the software and physical architecture to swing anything while maintaining control through rotation.

The movements I teach in my curriculum are for fitness, yet they're based on practical application. If you learn how to swing the mace in class, not only will you get stronger, but you'll develop the mindset and coordination to wield other weapons as well. My intention isn't to train soldiers—we're not fighting anyone but ourselves—but I won't say I wouldn't want my students by my side in the event of a zombie apocalypse, either.

Beyond work with unconventional weapons, the steel mace is a great precursor to train with a variety of tools. As it's got the longest lever out of the equipment you'll find in most gyms, it's going to be the hardest to control. It will help iron out any kinks in your joints. Your core will stabilize. Your balance will improve. Tools that are closer to you—everything that isn't the mace, in short—like the kettlebell and dumbbell, become far more manageable.

The importance of training with offset weight and rotational movements for sports can't be underestimated. Consider football: a receiver running downfield will have to turn and look over his shoulder to make a catch, but what if he's tackled while rotated? We're only prepared for what we practice, and in conventional sports training barbell squats and deadlifts alone don't prime an athlete for that type of load and impact. Swinging a mace, however, prepares for that eventuality, and builds the strength to maintain rotated positions without collapsing and sustaining injury.

Viking Ninja is all about longevity. Though most durability-specific exercises are performed with bodyweight (think yoga-like deep stretches), the mace is also a full-fledged durability tool. Using it unlocks tension in the shoulders, enabling movement through greater ranges. Once your brain "sees"—through pictures, video, or in person—the exercises you're expected to complete, it will constantly strive to move your body closer to the desired end range even if it isn't currently within your ability.

With this flexibility comes increased mobility. While flexibility involves passive improvement of range, holding a mace during moving means you will also build strength through your newfound potential. Flexibility (to a reasonable degree) is desirable in its own right, but part of durability is increasing resilience to injury. It only does so much good if your ankle can bend a little more before it snaps. What if it could support extra range and simultaneously fight the pressure of unexpected torque? While the mace most directly targets the upper body, moving through lunges and other positions improves mobility elsewhere.

This is why the mace is such an effective preventative tool for athletes and weekend warriors alike. There's no reason why your grandmother couldn't learn to use the mace —though a seven-pounder seems more appropriate than a twenty-fiver—to greatly improve her quality of life and chances of making it through a fall unscathed. We spend too much time worrying about performance and not enough considering what could go wrong. One injury and training comes to a halt—why not take time to improve both performance *and* resilience with a single tool?

Still, whether from an accident or due to negligence, injury will eventually happen if you're consistently pushing boundaries. But even if you aren't, what would you call the constant degradation in strength and structural integrity that comes from a sedentary lifestyle and poor posture? I would call it injury, and luckily the mace is just as powerful a restorative tool as it is preventative. Starting slow, the mace gradually reverses the poor posture that comes from atrophied muscles and connective tissue. All you need is to get started.

It's an unfortunate fact of life that most of us have lost connection to the basic patterns that underpin all movement: the squat, hinge, push, and pull. Chronic back pain, which so many people suffer from, is often a direct result of faulty movement. With proper instruction and conscious engagement, the mace is a didactic tool that will reestablish the patterns necessary for successful, pain-free movement in everyday life. It's not the only one that does this, but the scant stress it places on the body makes it ideal for both beginners and experts alike.

Two aspects of proper mace technique are most responsible for impacting posture. The first is the already-noted fact that it strengthens the shoulders and improves their mobility. Much of poor structure can be attributed to atrophied muscles of the scapulae, which results in hunched shoulders and a cascade of other problems. Virtually all elderly people have terrible shoulder mobility, and that extends to middle-aged adults as well. This problem is only exacerbated by the ubiquity of cell phones and computers. Poor shoulder range is a direct contributor to what we now refer to as text-neck.

The other part of the body that the mace heals so effectively is the spine. Many people unknowingly suffer from lordosis, an excessive forward curve of the lower back, or kyphosis, an exaggerated backward curve of the thoracic spine, both of which result in pain, impaired locomotion, and faulty alignment. Through reinforcing the basic movement patterns the steel mace strengthens the core musculature that lengthens and supports the back. The importance of this aspect to mace training can't be overstated, as deterioration of the vertebrae over time results in irreversible damage to the nervous system.

Inherent to rotation, a defining quality of the mace, is asymmetry, another often-overlooked element of training. Rarely do we receive or exert force linearly and from dead center, yet that is often exclusively how we train. In a barbell squat we move with equal load distribution, and it's the same with a push-up or pull-up. Yet with the mace we typically initiate motion from one side, which more accurately emulates movements like throwing a ball or punch, or even getting tackled from an odd angle. Strengthening both sides individually creates stable, dynamic strength.

In conjunction with this conventional lack of asymmetric training comes linearity. A squat, push-up, or pull-up only trains movement in a single direction. When running across a soccer field we cut in both directions, move up and down, twist, jump, roll. The mace is so valuable for athletics because of its stress on multi-planar movement. An athlete can only perform as well as he is trained, and moving in multiple vectors at once is key to effectiveness.

There are a number of reasons beyond the physical that make the mace such an effective tool. Some types of exercise are simply more engaging than others. Most people find it just about impossible to muster the willpower to go for a long run, but if you put a mace in their hands they can't resist the urge to swing it. Something about the tool is beyond motivating—it infects you with the desire to work.

Another key to long-term success is program adherence, and for all the aforementioned reasons the steel mace has a high rate of loyalty. This is partially because swinging a mace is downright sexy, and friends will flock to your side when you exercise. Nothing is better for adherence than a workout partner, and you'll have no trouble finding one. This is doubly important if you're a coach or trainer, as employing your mace with students is a terrific way to get them to love your training.

You can even tell your friends or clients this: with the mace, results are guaranteed. There are so many positive outcomes that it's impossible not to hit at least a handful of them. You can't swing the mace for an extended period without developing dexterity. Unless you've trained with the circus or are an accomplished gymnast, your range of motion is bound to improve. Many people are discouraged from starting programs because they believe they're bound to fail, yet as long as you pick up the mace you're destined to succeed.

The mace is particularly impactful for those interested in fighting, whether for sport or self-defense. The mace is fundamentally a weapon, and exercises like the 360, uppercut, or bayonet strike are combat techniques themselves. You don't have to be a soldier for self-defense skills to benefit you.

Most people interested in combat are stuck in their ways, married to one or two schools of thought. Swinging the mace broadens the horizons of any martial artist. It's common to take karate lessons as a kid or join the boxing club in college, yet few of us delve into the history of martial arts and their relation to fitness. The mace was not only

Viking Ninja Elements

used as a weapon, but also as a training method for wrestlers and warriors.

In kickboxing, the head is kept low while the shoulders are hiked to protect the chin from hands, feet, elbows, knees, and whatever else an opponent might throw at you. This results in unnatural tension around the neck, shoulders, and thoracic spine, which is aggravated by the particularly long hours most of these athletes spend training. The mace is an extremely effective tool for fighters, as it opens the shoulder capsule and relieves stress in surrounding areas.

Speed is typically avoided when weight training. You can certainly squat or deadlift explosively, and that's what olympic lifting is all about. But for most people, especially those without a great deal of skill and experience, speed under heavy load can be dangerous, particularly to the spine. With the mace, however, you can move dynamically through a variety of planes while remaining safe. Naturally you don't want to lose control and hit yourself, but you're at a much lower risk of ripping your joints around with an injurious degree of force.

On the opposite end of the spectrum, the mace is ideal for isometric exercises. Its offset weight challenges your body and stresses grip to the maximum. This is one area in which Erin Furry's Steel Mace Yoga truly shines. Depending on the routine, you can hold poses for any length of time, building and maintaining tension through a variety of ranges. This is particularly effective for building core strength and muscular endurance, though the applications are endless and can be bent to your goals.

Across this spectrum you will develop an understanding of static, fluid, and dynamic motion, which translates to all areas of fitness. The static element is the isometric component of Steel Mace Yoga, but it also comes into play during the general curriculum when moving slowly and locking in landmark positions. The fluid component is when you flow through exercises without stopping, while the dynamic involves accelerating and slowing down during various transitions.

It is through these tempos, ranges, and planes that you will grow to appreciate the immensity of human movement possibility. In daily life we're rarely challenged, as our routines are tame and pre-packaged. Once you begin to understand your potential with the mace you can begin designing your own routines.

Though it trains your central nervous system to communicate more efficiently with your muscular system, the mace also challenges your mind. It demands humility, as if you pick it up with a big ego you'll immediately be shut down. You can't start training with the mace for the first time and expect to swing a twenty-five pounder like it's nothing. Though even a forty-five pound bumper plate on the squat rack is relatively insignificant, mace weight is an entirely different animal.

The mace necessitates discipline through consistency and diligence. You may be pressed to rush, but taking things steadily is far more difficult. If you skip training days your skills will languish and your grip will weaken. A solid mace program requires that you work often but not too hard, at least in the beginning.

The tool breeds patience and builds character. You'll have to start slowly, focusing on technique and fine motor skills. With time they will translate to heavier weights, but without pacing yourself you risk injury or burnout. Still, it's much safer to train the mace with volume than most other tools. Regardless, be prepared to take your time and enjoy the journey.

Now, the mace is not a right, it's a privilege. As it's such a potentially devastating tool—how many thousands have lost their lives to them over the millennia?—we take safety very seriously. It's not a toy, and we stay within our abilities. If you can't follow those guidelines, don't pick up a mace. It's that simple.

NINJA

Opposite Viking and the steel mace is Ninja, which in the system represents bodyweight. It also equates to martial arts, which embody discipline through motion. The two aspects balance one another in countless ways, but the most important fitness connection is that before you can engage the steel mace or any other tool you need to have a firm understanding of your body and how to use it. Whereas Vikings always entered battle with a weapon and shield, ninjas were masters of minimalism, executing with the least amount of baggage possible. This necessitated that they hone their bodies like the sharpest of blades.

The reason Ninja is the concept behind bodyweight movement is simple: our aim is to move like a ninja. Being conceptual with your training gives it color and purpose—a target. The battle is just as much psychological as physical, and the clearer your goals, the better you'll perform. Just as we hope to emulate a Viking's raw power as he tears across the battlefield, we want to progressively become more fluid and seamless with our movements. This latter skill comes before the former, as you must be able to control your body with laser-like precision to complicate the situation responsibly with a mace, barbell, or any other tool.

To be a Jedi you have to manifest Ninja and Viking at the same time. It isn't enough to have one or the other and call it sufficient. You have to be strong with and without your weapon. But being a Jedi also means having a strong mind. Take Yoda, who has such a strong sense of right and wrong that he's literally able to control the external world with his mind. We can't do that—it *is* fantasy, after all—but the same principle applies. A strong mind can change the world. If you apply yourself anything is possible.

Both the Viking and Ninja elements of the system are rooted in philosophy, because knowledge precedes movement. Ninja is about understanding how to occupy your body rather than simply use your body. Anybody can get under a heavy barbell, grit their teeth, and force themselves to squat, but they're bound to get injured if they don't have sufficient prior experience.

Few people know themselves well enough to match their self-understanding to reality. Bodyweight movement is a way to venture deep into sensation and mindfulness. Our goal with Ninja isn't just to move better, but to foster a deep awareness of all the individual parts of our unique bodies and how they work together to form a whole. On any given day you have to know whether your ankle is ready for jiu-jitsu or if you have a slight tweak in your shoulder that could be further exacerbated by work with the bo staff.

To find discipline in movement we start slow. This is a journey we're embarking on, not a quick fix. Modern life has conditioned us to expect immediate gratification. We want movies at the click of a button, food hot and ready at our door after a phone call, and good health from twenty minutes on the treadmill. While technology may have made the first two possible, if you want to be strong and capable, it's going to take time and effort. From the moment we get up until we go to sleep we're constantly moving, but not in the right way. We're rushing to brush our teeth, to get to work, to scarf down donuts on our lunch break. To unlock our capabilities it's necessary to reject that, to slow down and find time for pure sensation.

Day by day we grow more blind to what's going on inside us. Ninja is so essential because it exposes the battle between you and yourself. Only you can feel your weakness, your fatigue, and the difficulty that comes from using your body properly during the search for ideal mechanics. That takes discipline.

We tend to go through our lives oblivious to all this. When we have joint pain we treat it with pills rather than searching for the root of the problem. If we can't sleep we don't consider the fact that maybe our bodies were meant to move for hours every day and that we have energy leaking from our pores. Instead, we treat insomnia with more pills, further dulling what languishing connection we have to our bodies.

Beginning this journey isn't without its pitfalls. We can't solve the problem of improving our health with the same level of thinking that got us into the predicament we find ourselves in now. That means killing the voice that tell us to rush and search for shortcuts.

With engaging Ninja comes responsibility—only moving through positions and ranges that are within your ability level. At the beginning, when you don't have the requisite sensitivity to your inner state, this means listening to your coach. Entering positions and ranges you can't maintain is how you get hurt and fail to learn the lesson you're trying to access in the first place. It means you lack the discipline to control yourself.

The ego is what tells us we don't need work, that we're already at the pinnacle of our existence. But none of us is at a hundred percent. We're all at step one, and there's so much room for improvement within the body—though naturally the mind and spirit deserve just as much attention. Ninja is about recognizing that there's ninety-nine percent of you out there somewhere just waiting for you to access it with the proper character and dedication. You'll find this through movement, which brings out humility by demonstrating that you're not as strong mentally, physically, or spiritually as you think you are.

It's impossible to reach that hundred percent, and that's the whole point of this endeavor. There are no limits other than the ones you set for yourself, and there's always room to grow. There's always more depth. You may think you've found the deepest kernel of yourself, but as you push further and harder you'll always find another level. There are no limits. You're as strong as you allow yourself to be, and Ninja is about pushing yourself to ever higher planes of performance.

Ninjas were trained to be the perfect assassins, and no one was more effective at execution, both literally and figuratively. Yet they didn't bow to their egos and suffer from excessive vanity. That ran counter to everything they believed in, to their very purpose. Ninjas never showed their faces. They didn't need to. They covered them up and let their actions speak. They were assassins. Their mission wasn't about praise and accolades, it was about performance. It's all about pride and the ego. You don't have to show your face, and you need to engrain that attitude deep in your being.

Though our philosophy celebrates Vikings and ninjas for their differences, they shared important characteristics, the most important one being that they were single-mindedly focused on task completion. But in this one uniting quality they differed in an important way—Vikings fought by day, whereas ninjas fought by night.

People say that ninjas hid in the shadow as if it were a

shameful thing, but that's not the way I look at it. They didn't fight *in* the shadows. They *were* the shadows. That's what made them so successful. No one could see them, and thus they were invincible.

You have to make your movement the same as a ninja's: effortless, silent, fluid. That's how you become untouchable. The goal is to perfectly execute your vision. You don't want hitches. There's no room for mistakes when your neck is on the line. It's just like the Jedi who understands the force within him—the Warrior Spirit—and can thus execute at the highest level whenever he's called upon. Once you condition that in movement, life outside the gym becomes easier.

You also have to admire their dedication and work ethic. Like Vikings, ninjas weren't royalty. They weren't special. They fought through the night but still had to work by day. They had a twenty-four hour battle. When they returned in the morning they had responsibilities for their family and villages. They were assassins in the first place because they needed money to provide. As with the Vikings, for whom brotherhood was imperative, you have to make your actions mean something not just for yourself, but for your community.

Even though Vikings fought in the light, they had a dark side. For ninjas that was an even bigger problem, since by their very nature they were already so close to the dark. There were times, for instance, when they were controlled by corrupt governments that didn't have the peoples' interests in mind. If you forget who you are and sell yourself to another set of principles you're committing spiritual suicide. Once you accept a philosophy or way of life, don't sacrifice what you believe in. It will rot your mind. Just because you operate in the dark doesn't mean you have to become the dark yourself.

It can so easily become kill, kill, kill without giving a care for people and their bodies. It's the same with training. You can fall into the trap of drill, drill, drill without paying attention to your health and wellness. Then you end up destroyed. Your structure breaks down and you injure yourself. You can't simply care about the sweat. You have to stay open to everything so you can make the right decisions and maintain awareness. Assassinate your ego, not your body.

LIKE WATER

Though Bruce Lee would have been the first to say actions speak louder than words, countless life-changing sayings have been attributed to him. The following is one of the quotes I come across most often, and it's deeply affected my own thinking, as well as the philosophy of the system I created:

"Don't get set into one form... Be like water. Empty your mind. Be formless, shapeless—like water. Now, you put water in a cup, it becomes the cup. You put water into a bottle, it becomes the bottle. You put it in a teapot, it becomes the teapot. Now, water can flow or it can crash. Be water, my friend."

This quote is ripe with all sorts of meaning. The following discussion isn't intended to be exhaustive or authoritative in any sense. I'm sure I hear different things in Bruce Lee's voice than you do.

The most powerful message I receive is that we must be adaptable in all things. There are times when we must be formless, yet there are also times when we must be rigid and unbending. Water has all of these capabilities, which makes it such a resilient material. If you can't be open-minded and flexible in a relationship, it will fall apart. But if you can't defend your positions in an argument you'll get stomped into the dirt. The wisdom lies not necessarily in accepting the truth to these words, but in learning when and how to apply them.

In Viking Ninja there are countless applications. Take bodyweight movement. First and foremost, our goal is to move fluidly, just like a ninja would slip through the shadows. If your squat, one of the foundational patterns, is jolting, then something's off. If you tried to do a double backflip and were hung up like that you'd land on your face. The ultimate demonstration of mastery is to move like water, to make it look effortless, and to have so much control over yourself that you can go as slow as humanly possible. Glaciers move with such power that they change the shape of the earth.

Though we may appear to flow, inside us is violence. Nothing about the activation in a double backflip is easy. If you're doing a pull-up properly, it shouldn't be easy either. But we control that crashing energy so that rather than manifesting as a hurricane it's a rapid river—or, as above, a slow, thundering glacier. We may be generating a tremendous amount of force, but we're controlling that output and directing it toward a specific end. It's aggressive but contained. We're roaring internally, but smooth in expression.

More abstractly, formlessness is an attitude. Your goal is to find balance. Lose yourself in the movement and become the movement. This stance results in the amplification of sensation and purpose as you cement the connection between mind and body. It can drastically improve your performance as you enter the mental state of flow.

A phrase I picked up at Onnit that I use often in this context is *make light heavy and make heavy light*. This usually applies more to work with tools, but the same principle applies to the body. When you're swinging around a light mace, you want to move slowly and with deliberate attention, focusing on your technique to make the mace as heavy as possible and thus get the most out of your training. But when you're swinging a heavy mace, you want to move as smoothly as possible to make the weight feel like a feather. It's all about emulating water.

It's also a matter of perception. People see a light mace and think nothing of it. Coincidentally, they probably haven't swung a mace before. But it doesn't take the whole ocean to drown you. A tiny glass of water can end your life just as quickly as the largest tidal wave. If you aren't careful a seven pound mace will break your body.

The same thing goes for the ocean and the heavy mace. The sea may seem calm, yet if you jump in and don't mind your energy levels you'll drown if you stray too far from shore. The currents could suck you down at any moment. Whenever you're training, even if you think you're in the comfort zone, maintain self-awareness and prioritize your safety. If you turn back to shore for a heartbeat you could miss the wave that's strong enough to snap your neck. People drown at the shallow end of the pool all the time. The water's not the one panicking, you are. Babies can swim, yet if you get pushed into the water and panic takes over, your composure goes out the window. We train to grow comfortable with fear, to let the Warrior Spirit guide our way.

Water can be tranquil and water can be rough. It can be formless or crashing. Neither state makes the water more or less dangerous—it's just different. We train to manifest that quality. It's our goal to be calm of mind yet capable of body, able to explode at an instant and accomplish whatever is necessary.

It's impossible to make that heavy steel mace float like a feather if you haven't mastered the light mace. That's where the ego gets involved. So many people walk into the gym and pick up the heaviest mace we have, squat all the plates they can fit on the bar, or simply compete with the biggest, toughest guy in the building. That's why they don't last long —they get hurt, beat up, humiliated.

It's tough enough to make the light mace heavy. Adaptation comes in stages. You don't start as water—that's the end goal. If we were already there, Bruce Lee's words would carry no meaning. It would be like suggesting that you try breathing.

The path to adaptability begins with taking your seven-pounder or ten-pounder and slowing things down to become effective and capable through all your ranges. Once you have those under your belt you'll be ready to handle the heavier mace, and your fluidity will already be there. If you've committed and set your intention, adaptation will come quickly.

Another aspect to the quote that I find extremely enlightening is the reference to cups and teapots. As I perceive it, having an empty cup or a full cup reflects the quality of being open or close-minded. In Viking Ninja we advocate for open-mindedness whenever possible. The system is not dogmatic. Naturally to be part of the community you must adhere to certain practices, but your being here is voluntary in the first place, and we would never say that there's only one way to do something. We do ask, however, that when people attend our certifications, workshops, or in some other way connect with our material they empty their cup and give us their due attention.

In general having an empty cup is positive. You never know what you'll learn. Having a permanently full cup is the sign of an overbearing ego, an unwillingness to listen to reason. But if you have an empty cup, you shouldn't fill it too quickly or else you're liable to spill the contents. This is what happens when someone tries to cram for an exam the day before and ends up making a mess of things: they take the test without having retained any of the information and consequently fail. What they should have done was attended each lecture and added a little bit to their cup every day. Slow and steady wins the race.

With Viking Ninja, we hope that our members will keep more than one cup. This is what I mean by dogma. There's no reason you can't be a martial artist, a yogi, and a ballerina all at the same time. The more knowledge you have and the more exceptional you are as a person, the more valuable you are both to yourself and the community. However, you should be careful not to discard the contents of one cup for another without due consideration. If fitness hasn't been part of your life for a long time, don't juggle ten cups, attending ten different schools every week. Rather you should take your time filling one before going to the next. Juggling is a great way to end up with shards of glass in your feet.

Within Viking Ninja we have cups for nunchucks, bodyweight, steel mace—there are plenty of them. You don't have to fill them all. You can pick and choose based on what suits you best. But for the cups you do choose to fill, it's necessary to maintain your discipline, dedication, and commitment by honoring the principles of the system. Without them you can't be like water. You end up flat and formless in all the wrong ways—you're a puddle, useless, a nuisance.

This quote isn't just abstract philosophy. I keep it in mind every day. It affects the way I perceive myself, certainly, but also how I approach the challenges I deal with everywhere I turn. When the burdens I carry are too heavy, I make them light. If I have to run a marathon, I'm going to run it one mile at a time. I'm not going to complain, dreading mile twenty-six before I even have my shoes on. Yet if my challenge is light, I'm going to make it heavy. If all I have to work with is a seven-pound mace, I'll move as painstakingly slow as possible, and I'm not going to put it down for an hour. I'll be shaking by the time it's over.

If you aren't challenging yourself, you're getting lazy. You're sinking. If you're sitting on your butt playing video games, stop. Work out. If you work out all day, stop. Go fishing. Whatever your normal is, break out of that mold. Find a challenge and surmount it.

CHALLENGE YOUR DISCIPLINE

Most of us have negative associations with the word discipline. It reminds us of getting punished in school, of being stripped of fun, of being told we were bad kids. Discipline means something different to me now, and a great deal of that comes from the fact that I'm imposing it on myself by choice. It's no longer an arbitrary thing clasped around my wrists like shackles by a prison warden I don't recognize.

Discipline comes down to honesty. If you say you're going to do something, you do it, and you do it to the best of your abilities. It's that simple. If you're not disciplined and you know it, stop being an imposter. Bring out the truth. There's a reason killing your ego and challenging your discipline go hand in hand.

Discipline means paying attention. It means staying focused. Being disciplined means doing what needs to be done. When given two paths, we're almost guaranteed to take the easy one. It's only natural. It takes something extra, a push from the Warrior Spirit, to make the hard choice and stay on that road, and it's what makes some people rise above the average to become exceptional. They put it in the work that others shrug off, and when they reach the apex of performance in whatever their field is the people who quit early say it was all luck. The application is where it gets difficult, and where the great separate themselves from the ordinary.

Discipline is also the level of self-expectation you carry everywhere in life. How you do one thing is how you do everything, and gains you make in one field will affect your performance elsewhere, if only because of the continually growing momentum of your mindset. If your ego is so huge that you can't hear or perceive the truth because it frustrates you, then you're not disciplined.

People grow weak because they can't control their emotions. Like a garden that doesn't get cared for, emotions go wild and start to rule over everything you do. Find a way to push yourself to the limits, walk out intact, and grow bulletproof to the chaos swirling around you in life that can override your self-control.

Embrace whatever triggers your emotional instability. You must learn how to own those triggers. Every battle starts in the mind, and after you win one, two, three battles you start to build velocity. It's like you have an internal suit of armor keeping you safe from everything that seeks to harm you. If political talk throws you off your game, then meditate for a few minutes and turn on the news. Immunize yourself to that stuff. If you can't survive the train ride to work without listening to a podcast or reading because the boredom is suffocating, cut that stuff out and relish the silence. Learn to make your mental state independent of everything outside it. This is exactly what we do in the gym to push past hurdles.

Things should never sidetrack the mind. You don't want mental warfare. Internal battle is far more stressful than punches to the body. When your mental state spirals out of control it can take a lifetime to heal. People will lose a leg and be back to running in six months like nothing happened, but if your ego grows too large and you get rejected on a date you might never recover.

In fitness, challenging your discipline means connecting your mind and body. When performing a given movement you have to be able to follow cues and hit landmarks despite fatigue or other sensations that make you want to fall apart. The gym isn't a place to gawk around or play on your phone. It's more than just a training ground for your body. Whenever you step through those doors you have to be turned on mentally.

Ninjas were the embodiment of discipline. They were assassins devoted purely to execution, both literally and figuratively. If they compromised anything in their mission, it could mean death. After all, they failed their ruler, who either paid them, owned them, or worked them in some other respect. Even if they survived the battle, they still had to answer to that higher power.

Being a ninja is all about organization. For them, challenging discipline meant being tactical. Your emotions, your ego, they want you to march forward without considering the consequences, because that's the easiest way to be. Yet that's how you get ambushed and make all the wrong moves.

Ninjas challenged their discipline by constantly perfecting their execution. No task could be completed swiftly or efficiently enough. There was no such thing as perfection, only excellence to ever greater degrees. To strive for excellence means being disciplined in practice to constantly seek improvement. The moment you think growth is impossible, either because your ego has poisoned you or you believe there's some sort of ceiling to your capacity, is the moment you fall back to square one. You've lost your Warrior Spirit.

Viking Ninja Elements

The Vikings were disciplined because they wanted to conquer—that was their goal—and they succeeded. They didn't assassinate like ninjas, but they executed. What's that if not discipline? They repeatedly made journeys across the sea that no one in the world thought was possible. No corner of Europe had any idea what was going on. For them, being disciplined meant thinking outside the box and doing the impossible, riding the tide of belief. If death wasn't enough to subdue their passion, then nothing was.

The Vikings won every battle, even if they lost. How? Because they did what they wanted, what needed to be done—the two were one and the same—and made sure they performed to their expectations regardless of the odds. If they retreated, it wasn't out of fear. It was tactical, like the ninjas. No one fled, because that would mean compromising the unit. If you were part of that army, you were there by choice. No one forced you to go.

Discipline is all about will, not compulsion. There's a major difference between discipline and tyranny. The first involves choice, the latter none. The former is rewarding mentally, physically, and spiritually, while the other only serves to break you down and make you submissive.

The Vikings challenged their discipline by constantly pushing toward conquest. No matter how many men died in battle, no matter how gruesome the war, the takeover, they didn't give up. They were disciplined to each other and their goals.

They were also disciplined *by* each other. Otherwise they would have failed. That's one reason brotherhood is so important to Viking Ninja. We feed off one other. If your friends are all hitting the gym to train, you're gonna be there. If your friends are lazy and playing video games instead, you're probably gonna do the same thing.

I walk into a gym and know immediately who has discipline and who doesn't. Who's chewing gum and blowing bubbles? Who's shouting on a headset? Singing? Mirror selfies? Flexing? Nowadays all I see is lacking discipline. It's just about having fun, being trendy, selfish, senseless, and calling out desperately for attention.

Where's the digging for depth? People stand around the gym digging for stuff that doesn't belong there, like Instagram followers. Are you trying to get stronger in body and mind? Or are you trying to grow a stronger social media presence? The gym has become a platform to fool the world into thinking you're something you're not. As soon as the cameras turn off it becomes apparent to anybody in the room that it was all a sham. It's all lies. That's not right.

You teach someone to challenge their discipline by giving them something new. You watch it affect them and then you determine where their head is. If they can't challenge themselves, if they give up too quickly, it shows a lot about their mental strength. It probably reflects where they are in life as well, because discipline translates from one pursuit to another. They're all related. If you always settle for less, you end up sinking. You never move forward. That's stagnation. Your life becomes a big stinking swamp.

Just as you challenge discipline inside the gym, you can do the same outside. Learn, grow, and apply yourself based on whatever you read or experience. Follow through on your knowledge. Listening and nodding is one thing, but acting is what really matters. We're defined by what we do and how we carry ourselves, not the lectures we sit through.

People who aren't necessarily the fittest demonstrate their discipline by showing up. My client Gordon Johnson is a perfect example. He's gotten strong as hell, but he's still heavy. His level of discipline is intense because he does a ton of work, and the more you weigh, the harder it is. He never gives up. He challenges himself by coming in, committing to excellence in his performance, following my instructions, and grinding through the discomfort. He's content with the training and never complains. And if he weren't that way, he wouldn't make progress and he'd never reach his destination.

If you don't stay dedicated, you get lazier. That won't serve you in any respect. You'll slide right back to square one. The following is a saying from one of the old sagas, the Vatnsdæla: "There is more honor in accumulating little by little than in reaching for the sky and ending up flat on your face." This idea harkens back to the importance of regression and progression in reaching progress. Too often we get greedy, listening to our egos, and grasp for too much too fast. That's how we get injured, and it's far more difficult to change your mind or spirit than it is to access your body. The wisdom in this proverb lies in accepting that though progress may be slow, it will be sure. When striving for any goal, settle at a pace that is sustainable. Don't bow to the ego and overshoot your capabilities.

YIN AND YANG

I always knew the Yin Yang would be a major part of my system. When Aubrey first called me the Viking Ninja, the clash of terms was so obvious. Could any two peoples be more different? Even the words are opposites. One is hard and the other soft. They were separated by centuries and thousands of miles, and yet they still somehow go together so well. They complement each other.

The Yin Yang is the same. It's a story of extremes that fit together like lock and key. Each of us has that in us. We're hot and cold, light and dark, brave and fearful. Without balance everything is chaos, yet we are each a complete person capable of amazing things.

In general, what the Yin Yang illustrates best is duality and the balance that any two opposing forces or ideas have to find if they aim to coexist in harmony. You can place any dichotomy on the Yin Yang and analyze why and how the two pieces sit there together. It has tremendous didactic potential if you use it correctly and responsibly.

Most obviously, you have white and black, or light and dark, and in Viking Ninja this begins in the center. We picture the Yin Yang as being located right in your core, and while the Valknut is more directly Viking-related, the Yin Yang pertains to Ninja.

The Yin Yang begins in the core because after we're conceived we start as a head and body, only for the limbs and appendages to emerge as we mature. The center is the starting point. Balance has to be there from the beginning. You don't find balance as you go along. When you step on a tightrope, you don't figure out balance halfway across. You better know what you're doing from the beginning or the whole operation falls apart.

The head and body always come as a pair. The Valknut is the head and the Yin Yang is the body. The Yin Yang balances them, as just having one on its own is meaningless. You need brain and brawn alike to be optimized.

Yet the body in itself must be balanced if you aim to understand it. Everything has to be in working condition if you want to control what you're operating. If one of your elbows is messed up, you won't be able to do a proper pushup, let alone any of the countless other fundamental movements in the Viking Ninja system. It's far harder to care for an imbalanced body than one that's running smoothly.

Of course, this is a process more easily discussed than performed. There are so many elements to consider when it comes to piecing together your unique puzzle. If you're constantly filled with adrenaline you're going to burn out. Cortisol? Chronic stress. You may not know the names for all the hormones, signals, and other things floating around your body that affect the way it runs, but you do have to become familiar with the sensations. Learning to right the ship comes with training and experience.

Perhaps the most obvious form of balance necessary for the body is energy intake and expenditure. This isn't a nutrition book, yet almost all of us have metabolic issues caused by unhealthy dietary habits. And you better believe that this leaks over into the mind. I'm not saying controlling it is easy, but acknowledging your lack of balance is the first step. Bridging those gaps will enable you to ultimately cross that tightrope toward optimization.

Balance isn't a static thing. If you look at the Yin Yang, it's full of motion. Light chases dark and dark chases light. Each is trying to swallow the other. We have that same tendency. It's so easy to lose control. The body wants you to listen to it exclusively, as does the mind. You can't let either one lose ground. They have to stay intact to keep the motion going. Otherwise one will eat the other, and it'll be a long road to untangle the confusion. Eventually it happens to all of us. If we experience a death or terrible injury everything can go out the window in the blink of an eye. You have to be most vigilant when you're most vulnerable.

But the black and white, the light and dark, the good and bad—they understand each other. Each side of a duality bears inherent respect for its partner. The Yin Yang portrays this with the tiny white circle in the black, the tiny black circle in the white. They are mirror images of one another, each containing a tiny piece of the other deep in its core. You can't have light without darkness or darkness without light. The concepts are intrinsically connected, and they cannot be split apart. If everything were good or everything were bad, there wouldn't be a word for either, as it couldn't carry any content.

The dark feeds off the light at its center, and the light feeds off the dark. But if the dark takes over completely there will always be that little seed of light at its core, which will eventually have to grow and capture back the positioning of the light. There's always that little failsafe. No matter how far gone you are, there's always hope to cling to. You can always recover. To me the Yin Yang is a symbol not only of balance, but of supreme hope.

The two forces keep one another in check. If you venture too far into darkness, the light will explode and bring things back to center. If you get too light, the dark will expand and swallow the light. Each side has its own agenda, but because they're in check they can't ever totally consume the circle. It's the perfect failsafe. Each side disciplines the other to maintain balance.

If your dark side is the intention to work out and improve yourself, you need light to slam on the brakes and keep you from sweating yourself to death or rupturing your muscles. The two result in progress, not burnout. The Viking Ninja Yin Yang is there to keep you fluid, not chaotic, and to maintain even distribution in all things so that your mind and body are capable of working together in a harmonious environment rather than allowing one to kill the other.

The Yin Yang also serves to balance the system itself and the archetypes espoused by Viking and Ninja. You have the black, the darkness of the Yin Yang, which is most often associated with ninjas, who fought by night and shadow. The light within them kept the task illuminated. It's the discipline that enabled them to execute, that showed them the path necessary for victory.

On the other hand you have the white, which represents the Vikings, who fought and traveled by daylight beneath that cold, white arctic sun. Yet the Vikings had darkness in them as well, and it propelled them to wage their wars, no matter how grueling or brutal they became. Light and dark utilize each other to succeed and maintain dominance in a harsh world. They may have been different people in different times, but they shared the Warrior Spirit.

I'm focused when I train, but in the back of my mind I always consider the Yin Yang, as balance is nowhere more important than when you're in the middle of execution. One false step, one trip-up, and you can injure yourself. The Yin Yang reminds me that my body and mind have to work together, that each one must be at a hundred percent to create a whole greater than its parts.

I put all of my intention into whatever it is that I'm doing, because if my energy is off and I lack the balance to perform, failure is inevitable. Failure can never be inevitable. You have to win every battle before you fight it.

I also keep the Yin Yang in mind whenever I approach a new tool or weapon. There's a lot of potential darkness in that situation. Sure, you may see the implement and hold it in your hands, yet there's way more lurking beneath the surface. If you pick up a calculus textbook, you may have a general expectation of what you're going to find, but you don't know a thing about the math. It's the same with the weight, rotation, technique, and science of a new tool.

You're going to experience all manner of insecurities and fear when doing something unfamiliar, but eventually the light will shine. Once you begin moving you'll surmount all that trepidation. Confidence will come as you perform. That small light circle is the knowledge of where you'll be in the future as you continue to progress through the unknown, while the darkness in the light reminds you of the need to continue your practice and never forget or discount that which you already know. The two are tied together and can never be cut apart.

This is the attitude I take toward nunchucks. It's how I approach the bo staff. It's how I approach any new weapon or tool in my practice. With striking, it becomes your hands rather than an external object. It never ceases to amaze me how we're blessed with these amazing bodies, and yet for all our years and experience there's so much we don't know about how to use them. The Yin Yang reminds me of that and keeps me curious, prepared to explore when I enter the gym and design new training methodologies or delve into those created by others.

Whenever I undergo that type of endeavor, I make sure to respect the darkness. Otherwise you can get squashed fast. It's also where fear grows. You can't be overly fearful, nor can you be too brash. It's all about that healthy medium of respect. If you're too cautious, you may ignore the unknown entirely, only sticking with the light. Then you'll never learn anything new and never progress. But if you dive head first into the dark, you might not come out. You might get injured or simply frustrated by the difficulty. Be wary of your ego and be wary of your insecurities. Take a flashlight when you go cave-diving. You need to know where you're going. Yet you'll go blind if you stare at the sun for too long. It's complex, but that's why we use the Yin Yang. It reminds us of the simplicity in all things.

There are so many important dichotomies to navigate in life. To get pleasure, you need pain. Neither works without the other. They're tied together. If you experience one, you have to remember that the other is waiting for you on the flip side of the coin. Don't get comfortable with pleasure, because pain is coming, but don't lose hope in pain, because you'll soon find your release. To go to heaven you need to go through hell. If you sell your soul to the devil, it may be sweet at first, yet you'll spend a long time in fire and brimstone as payment.

People always want the light first. That's because they're impatient and discount their future selves. But you have to be calm and considerate. Maybe it will be easier to bite the bullet now and relax later. You'll certainly be saved plenty of anxiety. It's also not always about what comes first. Everything depends on the situation. Be humble. Don't start the race with a sprint—end that way so you make sure you've given it your all. If you follow your heart, chances are you'll make the right decision. Follow the path and be disciplined. Ego throws off balance. Stay humble and you'll find the light.

Perhaps the most important lesson the Yin Yang teaches involves relationships. We all have a tendency to think about ourselves before anyone else. It's natural. We only feel our pain directly, our hunger, our desires. Yet if you want to have healthy relationships, if you want friends and loved ones, you have to meet in the middle. If you aren't equally satisfied, there's no balance and the relationship can't work.

The same concept applies not just to individual relationships, but to those that make up a community. Everything has to be in balance or else it will fall apart. If one person tries to hog all the attention, he'll be cast away. If one faction's values change, the Yin Yang will splinter and the duality will no longer exist. If one aspect of the community begins to do damage, whether through competition, dishonesty, or some other misalignment of intention, it swallows up everything that's good in the group, compromising it and ultimately destroying the brotherhood. At that point it may be easier to salvage that which is still there and start something new rather than attempt to rebuild the wreckage from the inside out.

Balance can be thrown off by the smallest things, which is why organizations are often so fragile, and which is why I'm being so careful to establish the values of Viking Ninja from the beginning. I want to make sure it's clear to everyone from the onset what we stand for and what our goals are.

BODYWEIGHT

Bodyweight movements play a huge role in Viking Ninja. Despite all the philosophy, this system is first and foremost about fitness. In my experience, few gyms give this type of exercise the attention it deserves. When most people work out they may do a set of push-ups. They might even give pull-ups a try. Crunches are a mainstay, but that's the end of the list. If they aren't chained to a treadmill, they'll make their way to the machines—or, if they're adventurous, the free weights.

This picture is all wrong. Before you work with tools you have to engage your hands, feet, hips, shoulders, and every other part of you. Bodyweight anchors movement Viking Ninja. You have to understand the patterns that underlie all motion. You need the fundamentals, and very little of it is conscious.

Your subconscious will come to grasp the axes, the mathematics, the science, and how it all mixes together to keep you safe and efficient in motion. Only once you have a firm grasp on all of these foundational skills and your nervous system has a basic level of intelligence should you begin to work with tools and the more advanced elements of the system. Regardless of whether you follow our programming, it would be wise to heed this reasoning the next time you visit a gym. What business do you have bench pressing four plates if you can barely do ten push-ups with proper form?

That being said, philosophy is a major part of bodyweight. Why are you moving in the first place? That's a big question. Hopefully if you're reading this book you don't need to be convinced that fitness is important for a fulfilling life. Provided you understand its significance, you then need to commit and dedicate yourself to that practice.

Bodyweight is an example of discipline in expression. Forget freedom when you're getting started. You need to iron out the basics. There are countless potential movements, but you have to walk before you can run. You've seen ninjas in movies do all sorts of acrobatics, and you've seen gymnasts do the same. I promise you that they all started with the basics. If you asked any of them to bang out some pull-ups, they'd murder rep after rep without a thought. They could crawl across the room in twenty different ways, return in another twenty, and then balance on their hands til the sun sets.

When you begin a new practice you have to respect the basics. If you're picking up a basketball for the first time, you don't work on your cross-over, you just dribble the ball while standing still. With bodyweight the corollary is balance, as you need to be stable if you hope to move safely and effectively. When balance becomes your priority, the path to progress grows clear. Once you can perform a substantial amount of volume in any particular movement while maintaining your structure and activation, you can move on to a more advanced progression.

Discipline comes in adhering to the cues and requirements of an exercise. It also comes in the form of patience, as we all want to skip ahead to the fancy things as quickly as possible. That, however, is a good way to get hurt. The foundations earned their name for a reason—without them, whatever lies above collapses. A one-armed handstand comes after a two-armed handstand, and running comes after walking and crawling. No baby ever sprinted out of the womb. Not even Usain Bolt.

Though it's a gateway to the steel mace, weapons, and training with other tools, bodyweight is extremely important in it's own right. Sometimes you have nothing to use but your hands and feet. You can't carry a steel mace in your back pocket when you're walking home late at night. What if someone's chasing you and you can't hop over a fence or crawl under a car? Being a master of your own body is not only necessary for that type of situation, but it is key if you want to call yourself a fully fledged human being. We neglect our bodies just as much as we do our minds, and the sad fact of the matter is that most of what you see people doing in the gym doesn't help them overcome either limitation in the slightest.

If your bodyweight movements are terrible, you have no business picking up a mace or kettlebell. You have to understand how to rotate and activate your supporting musculature. As soon as you put a tool in your hands, which complicates the physics, what little form you do have will fly out the window. That steel mace is going to own you. Your structure will crumble.

If you were a Viking, that mace would be worth less in your hands than on the ground, as you wouldn't be able to generate enough force to deal a blow or protect yourself from one. At least you could run faster if you weren't holding it. Bodyweight is the safest way to learn how to move, as you don't have external load that could harm your body or exacerbate any pre-existing and unaddressed conditions.

Part of what makes Ninja so powerful is that it gives the Warrior Spirit something to imitate. Regardless of what may or may not have happened five hundred years ago, everybody's seen movies and has an idea of how ninjas moved.

That's the exact type of weightlessness we want to emulate when we do our bodyweight work. It should look effortless, free, and powerful. Now, will it always feel that way? No. Fitness shouldn't be easy, but if you're moving fluidly you're on the right track. The math lines up. Your physics are on point. You never perform better in the real world than you do in practice, so when you're training you always need to shoot for perfection.

If we're training to move effortlessly, then just like the ninja you have to focus on execution. That means being disciplined with your dedication to the practice. You're not at the gym for fun. You're not here just to break a sweat, either. Everything has a purpose. Keep your body intact. Use tactics. This philosophy is heavy, and revolves around reason. With every rep you do and every breath you take, you need to struggle toward your goal, which is improvement, moving better than you did the last rep, better than you did the day before.

Bodyweight training will translate to every sport you play, every physical activity you engage in. Every day your body undergoes stress, and we train to counteract those forces and grow stronger. We're imbalanced, sick, torn, emotionally wrecked. At the end of most days we're in survival mode, though we rarely think about it that way because we're so used to it. With bodyweight training we aim to raise our strength level and contend with everything life throws at us. We want to understand the human body and how to pace it. Movement should be your stress-release valve. It should free you from the emotional baggage you rack up every day.

In all sports you're dealing with adrenaline and getting gassed up, but different activities require different types of energy. You're either working in short intervals or for long periods of time. In football, for example, you have intervals. Set, hike, boom. The play is over. It's like that every time. Soccer, on the other hand, is totally different. Aside from substitutions every once in a while, the game just keeps going. There are two forty-five minute halves. Some players will be in for the whole game, and they're going to make it look easy.

I want my athletes able to do both. That's the type of bodyweight I'm looking for. We have to strive for that. I want to see where the human body can go. I want to see people exceed their limits. A hundred thousand years ago we may not have been kicking balls around or scoring touchdowns, but we may as well have been because it couldn't be more obvious that we were designed for these things. If we're committed to the practice, we're going to succeed.

Unfortunately, however, we're almost all broken. We evolved to do these crazy things, but we've failed our blueprints. The goal of Viking Ninja is to take anyone, no matter their state, and through steady, disciplined training reach that pinnacle of performance that once seemed unthinkable. The next step is to exceed even that, and then to keep going. There are no limits. Everyone should be equipped with the physical strength to contend with life and the trials it brings.

Bodyweight also plays a major role in the martial arts. We all have to be versatile and adaptable, and a predictable fighter won't last long. Part of battle is having a wide range of abilities so that no one ever knows what's coming. Movement patterns apply everywhere. Push-ups aren't about doing push-ups. They're about catching yourself if you fall down in a tennis match or are controlling an opponent underneath you while wrestling.

Jiu-jitsu, for instance, is all about movement strategy. You must be able to manipulate both yourself and your opponent if you want to get the kill. You need to be able to move in a wide variety of patterns, whether that's on your back or on top, rolling around or standing up.

The following principle of Onnit's teachings is simply another way of explaining the idea behind Ninja and bodyweight movement. The United States Special Forces has a phrase used often around the Onnit Gym: *Slow is smooth. Smooth is fast.* John and Shane put their own spin on it by saying: *Slow is smooth. Smooth is beautiful.* Above all other metrics, form is the most important at Onnit and Viking Ninja.

Training bodyweight enables people to leave their sport and engage in different patterns that will translate back to what they're used to doing. You better believe I take NFL athletes through the same movements I'd go through with a UFC fighter. It's all about connecting the mind and body. I want to open my athletes' minds to their capabilities, to open their bodies to new ranges that will leave them more effective in their chief pursuit.

All of our sensory systems compute differently. You have to connect your hands and feet, your knees and elbows, your hips and shoulders. The more experience you have, the better your body is at moving. You'll need less conscious awareness in the moment, and yet you'll move more safely and efficiently, reducing the incidence of injury.

Viking Ninja bodyweight isn't just push-ups. It's not just squats. There's a whole range of different movements geared toward taking you through all the complexities of life, which is rarely linear like a push-up or squat. We're twisting, engaging multiple muscle systems, moving at different paces that require different levels of activation in different structures.

Viking Ninja Elements

We focus on the details to make sure everything is as clean as possible. I don't tolerate laziness in myself or others. You shouldn't tolerate it either. Your goal should be to seal every leak of strength. No matter what you're doing, the entire body should be at work. Your brain needs to know how to use your hands and feet and everything in between.

Learning that it's all about the mind requires going through a rite of passage. You have to be shown that your mind and body are disconnected. If you put someone through a grueling workout and they quit, they'll tell you it was their cardio, not their willpower. Your body is the one telling the truth—the mind gave up on it. You have to dig yourself out of your own ditches. There are no scapegoats in real life, and especially not in fitness.

HONOR YOUR DEDICATION

"Live through your Warrior Spirit and honor your dedication." Those are the words written on the shield in the Viking Ninja sigil, and if I get plenty of questions asking what the sigil itself means, I get just as many about the runes. It says something about the state of both honor and dedication in today's world that the idea is so foreign to most of us.

To honor your dedication means two things in concert. The first is understanding the commitment you're making when you accept the mission to constantly exceed your limitations. The second is in doing so realizing that it's unwise to overwhelm yourself with a weighty decision or course of action that you're going to regret later.

Dedication means sticking to your beliefs and goals in the face of hardship. We honor that commitment by remembering our passion and never letting it die. Life is meaningless without dedication. If you wander with the wind you're little more than a bacterium or virus, feeding off whatever you land on. You're fungus. There's no success because there are no challenges. You're apathetic, and if you're possessed of apathy you may as well be dead. Drive, desire, inspiration: these are the things that distinguish us from dust.

Dedication is what pushes you to the next level. If you're a lifelong athlete, at some point or another injury will occur. Dedication gets you through it. Marriage, family, relationships—nothing worthwhile comes easy, but when we believe in something we press through the tough times. This is a daily thing. You honor your dedication rain or shine, and every time you persist through pain your dedication grows stronger.

This also means self-respect. So many of us hate ourselves. We look in the mirror and wish we were something else. We have terrible relationships with our friends and family, our work, our bodies. Honoring your dedication means committing to improve those aspects of your life. They're all you have.

When we're not dreading the future, we look back at the past and only see regret. That's the opposite of how you should live. Every day you need to make choices you can be proud of in the future. This is the type of life that lets you sleep well at night, and it requires reflection. You have to look back on your past, starting with where you began, and evaluate the journey. Did you give it your all along the way? Did you accomplish everything in your power? You have to understand these things, or otherwise you're liable to leak energy and strength. Self-respect, just like dedication, is a self-fueling engine. When you believe in yourself you're going to push harder and longer.

Honoring your dedication also means respecting others, not just yourself. You have to honor your peers and teachers. You have to respect the process, the drawing board. It means following and accepting progressions and regressions and how they fit into the system.

It's important to be supportive of others, but be careful

of what you're supporting and how you're doing it. All your actions are a reflection of your character and the beliefs you aim to espouse. What you support must be worthy of your philosophy.

I honor my dedication to my teachers by practicing their templates the way they were intended. It's my responsibility as a student to make an attempt to understand my teachers' intentions for how and why anything should be done, and I do this by reproducing their techniques with the highest possible fidelity. No teacher wants their work to be forgotten. When I perform anything I've learned, I ask myself whether or not my teacher would accept what I'm doing. Would they be proud? That tells me a lot about whether I'm in the right place.

Once you accept a teacher, you must see them through. That's not to say you won't make mistakes, nor that they won't. My personal history with the steel mace is a good example. I engineered the curriculum for mobility, strength, restoration, and rotation. If you go outside of that before mastering the basics, I can't be held responsible for the outcome. It's great to be creative, but I researched, trained for years, and failed, failed, failed. It was all to create something. This is the process any good teacher goes through, and it's how they're able to transmit refined knowledge to their students. Respect that effort by giving the work the consideration it deserves rather than beginning to make changes and modifications right off the bat.

People try to be different for its own sake, but they have to understand that if the science isn't there, if the math doesn't make sense, then what they're doing isn't fitness. It isn't training. There will be no results, and any outcome will be negative for the body. Anyone can pick up a kettlebell and spin around in circles with it, but where's the "training" in that? Nowhere, as far as I can tell. It may be an exercise in dance or creative expression, yet it doesn't have a meaningful effect on strengthening the mind and body, especially not compared to the kettlebell training of a master like Eric Leija at Onnit.

My steel mace work relies upon radiation to strengthen the nervous system with a long-levered, offset tool. It makes things harder rather than easier. That's the goal of training. Why makes things easy for your body? That's play, not training. It does your body no service. If your aim is strength and power throughout life, then you can't play—you need science. I can't speak for any other curriculum, but what I do know is that if you're dedicated to the craft you will find amazing results.

To honor the process means following the progressional steps. It won't serve you to skip the basics and go straight to the most advanced movements. That's not honoring your dedication—it's spitting on your dedication by trying to skip the grind and look cool for the cameras. You can't cheat strength. You don't go from addition to calculus, nor do you go from recess football to the NFL. All growth begins with a seed. First come the roots, and in time you will have a flower. Some grow at different speeds, but even the fastest will need to have patience.

You can't force a plant to grow quicker, though you can nurture it. If you try to force your own growth, you're not committing to patience and you miss out on the whole progressional process, which is crucial not just for your body but for your mind. Do you want to be injured? Do you want to make irreparable mistakes? That's what happens when you go too fast and get caught up in confusion.

Injuries don't last two days. If you hurt your spine, it'll take a year before you're back to normal. A wilted flower may push hard to grow fast because it's desperate and panicking. It may believe it's winning, beating the other flowers, but sooner or later it'll topple over to the dirt when its stem can't support the weight any longer.

To honor your dedication you have to know where you're committing yourself, why you're doing it, and how you will be rewarded—whether it's a purse for winning a fight or the rush from sealing a business deal. You can't be dedicated if you don't have a path. Purpose must precede all action, or else you're little more than an animal, motivated only by the chemistry of pleasure.

Accomplishment, success, results—those are the goal. Yet why are they significant? You have to be sure of yourself. You have to believe in what you're doing. If you don't, it's time to sit back and reevaluate the direction you're going in life. Better sooner than later, as there are few things sadder than an old person looking back on their deathbed at everything they did and realizing they were never happy, that their life had no meaning.

Once you find your purpose, once you realize what you must do, your dedication can't only be fifty percent. You have to be all-in. Otherwise, why do it? You aren't living life to the fullest. Make your commitment a hundred percent every minute of every day. We only live one life, and there are no repeats. Every day is final. The upside is that tomorrow is anything but determined. You can wake up and make it whatever you want. Even if yesterday was wasted, the future is yours if you're willing to reach out and take it.

Dedication and fitness go hand in hand. There's no more readily apparent evidence of dedication than how you take care of your body. And the way this dedication becomes visible is by realizing the ultimate goal of fitness in killing the ego. Anything that detracts from that has to be discarded.

Dedication means working through the good times and the bad with the same resolve. The problem—or blessing—

of pain is unavoidable. You have to be prepared for it. There will be discomfort in your journey. How can you expect to knock down walls without breaking a sweat?

Still, you need to take your body where it's never been before in the safest possible manner. We draw upon dedication to push past anything that tries to hold us back. Living through your Warrior Spirit will take you farther than any idea ever could.

Honoring your dedication means respecting the commitment you've made not only to training, but to everything you do. Your life, your house, your body—they don't make messes on their own. You're the only agent in the situation. You make the mess.

Treat your home with respect. Treat your tool with respect. Treat your body with respect. They give you strength. You have to respect the atmosphere you inhabit, or otherwise you only end up harming yourself. If your atmosphere begins to deteriorate, the energy of the situation will go downhill. Keep things intact. Respect your gym like martial artists do their dojo.

Vikings honored their dedication to each other. They would avenge the fallen and fight to the last man. Ninjas honored their dedication to a specific task. If you have community and goals, then you win. If you add discipline to rugged strength and grit, you win. Organization and effectiveness? Takeover. Warrior Spirit and dedication? Victory.

THE VEGVISIR COMPASS

The Vegvisir Compass is another symbol integral to the philosophy of Viking Ninja. Along with the Yin Yang and the Valknut, it forms the basis for finding and acting on your Warrior Spirit. A thousand years ago the Vegvisir Compass served as a protective rune that if worn by a Viking would enable him to survive rough weather without getting lost. No matter how brutal the conditions, if he had the compass and his heart was pure he would always reach his destination safely.

If you have the Vegvisir, wherever you go, no matter what path you take, you'll never be lost. That's why the compass was so powerful for the Vikings. When they set out to sea, who could say what they'd encounter? Navigation was so rudimentary back then that it was impossible to know where—or even if—they would land.

The Vegvisir solved that problem. No matter where they struck shore, they knew what to expect—and that was victory. It was all mental, all self-belief. They didn't just hug a token and hope for the best. It was about hard work and brotherhood. The Vegvisir was just the reminder, the symbol of their effort, and with it came the knowledge that it would all pay off in the end.

When you set forth to achieve any goal, whether it's getting a black belt, curing cancer, or passing high school chemistry, the stars have to align. You have to get your mind-bind right. You have to balance your efforts with recovery. You have to keep your discipline intact and remain dedicated to the task. The mental game is all about the Valknut, whereas the Yin Yang provides you balance. Once you have both of those, you've found your Vegvisir Compass, and that means you can't fail. You have all the prerequisites to survive and navigate the path.

If you've connected mind and body, your heart is ready to lead the way. The Valknut is the mind and the Yin Yang is the body, but drive and passion lie in the heart with your Vegvisir. Passion tends to wane—and quickly—once hardship is encountered. After untangling your mind with philosophy and balancing your body through maintenance work and movement, if you're strong enough to keep your discipline alive then your heart is ready. I will always support you, Viking Ninja will always support you, and you can never be lost.

Even if you begin to stray from your path, the community will help you. An aligned mind, a balanced body, and a pure heart work like the strongest magnet. No one will forget you, no one will leave you, and everyone will want to be part of your journey. When we see the Warrior Spirit, we may not have the name at hand for what we're looking at it, but it's the most attractive thing a person can possess.

The Vegvisir means a lot of things to different people, and it's not my place to tell anyone how they should perceive it. Some think the rune truly possess power, whereas others see it as a symbol. No matter how you look at it, this latter point must be true. Keep the image close to your heart as a reminder that if you respect the concepts you've learned and the training you've been through, you have all the preparation needed to succeed. You don't need magic to survive and thrive—all you need is yourself, the best self you can be.

If you don't use your mind and body efficiently, the compass is going to disappear. You have to be focused. You have to constantly exceed your limits. The Vegvisir isn't a given—it's a privilege you must earn and hold onto with a tight grip. Once you get it you don't let go—that defeats the purpose. Once you get onto the path, why would you step off? Never go down without a fight. Never lose the fight within. You're always at battle, and that's what the Warrior Spirit is all about.

That's why when I wake up I don't like to think I have the Vegvisir. I won't wear it on my body. I have to earn it each and every day to show I'm fighting to be on the path. You can't expect anything to be given to you. That's how you fail. That's how you decay. Now, after I've worked my mind and body, after I've demonstrated to myself that I'm worthy, that I've battled to exceed myself, then I'm ready to wear the Vegvisir because it tells me I've won the day and am only going to keep on crushing. I'm riding the path like it's a wave. But if I lose momentum, if I forget myself, you better believe that compass is coming right off. It always has to be earned.

Just because I don't wear the compass in the morning or before I train doesn't mean I don't have a path. I know that path, and you have to be confident in it if you want to succeed. Being all about heart, the Vegvisir feeds on self-assurance.

You can have multiple paths. The Vegvisir has runes shooting off of it in all directions, because no matter which way you turn you're going to find the way. I have to be a father, a teacher, a husband, a coach. I have to care for myself, too. There are countless directions in which I have to travel—in which we all travel—but underlying it all is the necessity to believe in yourself. And if one path changes, if one path ends, there's always the others. There are infinite paths to travel, and you can never fail. Take one road until it ends, and then find yourself on the next.

The nature of the mind is to be chaotic. It's scrambled up ideas and emotions. Yet if it can be balanced through the Yin Yang, then the Vegvisir will give it direction. Just as everyone's mind is different, their balance will look different, and so in turn will their compass. None of us travels the same path as anybody else. If you want to be the best bowler in the world, that's awesome, but it's not the direction I'm heading in. The Vegvisir leads in every direction, and they all point toward fulfillment. It simply looks different for each person.

The Vegvisir played an important role in Ninja. Once ninjas found their discipline, they were ready to execute their mission. They had to stay balanced both in combat and flight. For tasks that were so tight, there could be no disorder. The compass is the through-line for all of that. No matter what path they were sent on, they executed.

The Vikings, on the other hand, were all about the mind. No matter what they had to do physically, even if it meant facing death in battle, their mind carried them through. The Vikings thrived on chaos. Odin, or their belief in him and the afterlife, gave them that power. That mindset took away all fear of failure. No matter how it ended, they won. If they died in battle, they won. If they lived to fight another day, they won. That's the definition of the Vegvisir Compass. Every path was the right path, because they were never afraid of what they'd find. It was always victory.

Ninjas were so balanced that they could go anywhere

and execute, whereas the Vikings were so strong-minded that no matter where they went or what they did they succeeded. If we can take both of those qualities, balance in body and strength of mind, then we have achieved true excellence and unlocked the key to the Warrior Spirit, which means that no matter where we go we will be on the path.

People come to me all the time without their lives in order. They don't know what their path is. Some don't even know they should be looking for a path. They're out of shape. Maybe they're not working or they're stuck at a dead-end job. They all ask for advice.

They want you to show them the way, but that's not how it works. You can't just give someone the compass. It's not something you hand out or buy at a store. We all have it. It's deep inside us, and it can be hard to find, but it's there. Anyone can access it. The way you take it out is by living through your Warrior Spirit. If you lose the Vegvisir you can get it back, but it will be hard.

This starts with belief. You have to believe in yourself and what you're capable of, which is why the body is such a powerful tool. In the gym you find that self-belief by challenging yourself to overcome perceived limits. You can't do a push-up? Well, do what I tell you and I promise we'll get there in a couple of weeks. Once those victories start mounting you begin to understand, and that's the first step to finding the Vegvisir, because that self-efficacy will extend beyond the gym to the rest of your life.

As coaches and trainers, that's what we do with our lives. We know. I know. I've done it a thousand times. People who don't think there's a path for them are dead wrong. We all have one. It's just a matter of putting the time and effort into exploring yourself. After finding that self-belief, there's a whole other set of steps and protocols to excavating your compass, yet because it's different for everyone it can't so easily be written about. First you need confidence.

MARTIAL ARTS

The martial arts are essential to Viking Ninja. I'm not talking about the schools you find on every corner with students lined up in rows bowing to their senseis. There's nothing wrong with that, provided the business is reputable and the teachers knowledgeable, but with Viking Ninja the martial arts are meant to teach you how to master your body and discipline your mind through fitness.

Vikings and ninjas both had their martial arts. Those of the former were never formally written down, but based on treatises from surrounding times and cultures, as well as testimonies of the conquered, the Scandinavians were more than simply adequate with their tools, and were extremely adept both with weapons and hand-to-hand combat, particularly wrestling. Ninjas, however, drew from a wide variety of Eastern practices.

When you combine the two types of warfare into one system, what you have is no longer traditional. Our goal isn't to bow down before arbitrary rules, but to take what works and discard the rest, seeking only to become the best. Here I like to think of Onnit's pillar, "Unity in Diversity."

I don't care who created something, whether it's a tool or body of knowledge—if it works, my aim is to integrate it into the system and build something beautiful with it. Take nunchucks, for example, which I've given a Viking approach by stressing the development of power through focus. As far as I'm concerned, the nunchucks are no longer about fighting, but instead about fitness and strengthening the mind and body. The weapon becomes a living thing dedicated to teaching control, new movement patterns, and the dexterity to direct an unwieldy, resisting implement.

Training in the martial arts with Viking Ninja isn't necessarily about combat, but the other elements of fitness it will bring you. To defend yourself you will need to learn footwork, proper movement patterns, and a whole panoply of skills, all of which will return you to the principles of Viking Ninja by strengthening your ability to pay attention, harness your dedication, and improve your discipline.

Just as your body grows reactive and capable, your mind will sharpen. Movements that were once chaotic become dynamic but controlled. This will translate into the rest of your life as decisions grow more solid. We're all slaves on some level to the monkey mind, which runs wild whenever we try to calm ourselves, and being able to control your body through a wide range of movement enables you to redirect that focus inward and conquer the thoughts that won't leave you in peace. Martial arts serve to blow away the smog that suffocates a clouded mind.

The simple fact is that without developing attention you won't be able to improve. The two processes go hand in hand. You can't perform at a high level while thinking about things that don't bear on the moment. When Michael Jordan was in the throes of a championship game his mind was on nothing but the hoop. It's the same with Cody Garbrandt in the ring or Lance Armstrong when he was on his bike. And if you take something like the martial arts that require such a demand on your fine motor skills, you have no choice but to batten down the hatches and execute.

Not only do martial arts clear away the fog, they tighten the wires that connect mind and body. For so many of us there's a huge gap between how we think we move and reality. This is brought to light by mirrors or film, and it's why few of us like hearing our voices recorded or seeing pictures of ourselves. Martial arts training makes movement clear and seamless. We were all born with a tremendously sophisticated movement apparatus. The only hitch is that it's atrophied from so much disuse. The patterns we were born with will rise up out of the murk.

Finding newfound abilities breeds confidence, and yet Viking Ninja is about never having to fight if you can avoid it. Still, that discipline will turn you into a lethal weapon any way you look at it. No longer will you need to fear confrontation if you lack courage. At the end of the day it's still martial arts. Whether you're working with your bare hands, the nunchucks, or the steel mace, you'll be able to defend yourself against anything that comes your way.

This self-assurance extends beyond the physical. We fear our bosses, we fear failure, we fear not being able to put food on our plates or those of our family members. We all have different pasts, different things that have beaten us into submission, but it comes down to a deep-seated belief that we are inadequate and unable to produce, unable to enact meaningful change in our lives.

Martial arts teaches you about the power you have within that's waiting to be let out. We all have the capacity to be terrifyingly effective. Understanding this will enable you to escape the fear that's holding you back. You'll grow strong enough to express yourself, to take what you deserve, to love yourself for the person you are and not hate yourself for the person you wish you were.

Yet the outcome isn't vanity. It's not ego. The martial arts train humility, not violence. Destruction is the dark side. We don't use anything we learn against other people unless it's to protect ourselves. The worst thing in life you can be is a bully, preying on those unable to defend themselves. That's cancerous, and the opposite of the Viking Ninja way. We aim to help others, to lift them up to a higher level with us, to share what we've learned.

Self-love is only one of the virtues brought on by martial arts training and learning to master yourself through the pursuit of a difficult passion. Above almost all other activities, martial arts will teach you patience. Learning to strike, to defend yourself, to wrestle or swing a weapon, requires time. It will take years to master the finer points of technique, to train your body to work in concert with your mind. If you're dedicated, you will need to learn patience, or else you'll drop like a fly.

The martial arts will show you where you lack discipline. If it's your first day with the nunchucks and you get frustrated, you didn't start with the right mindset. I promise you you'll swat yourself in the wrist a few times. Maybe even your face. But if you throw the nunchucks across the room and storm out, what was it all for? Your commitment was weak.

You have to show empathy for yourself. You're relying on your ego, which is telling you to get it done and prove something. But you have nothing to prove. You're a beginner. It's your first day. This is something that needs to be celebrated, not lamented. You should be proud of yourself for taking the initiative. It's an exciting time. You've accepted your potential, and you should enjoy the journey rather than watch the clock for every second that passes.

If you hit yourself, stumble, or otherwise make a mistake, be content with that. It's part of the process. Keep going forward and you'll find success. If you're kicking bags, you'll scrape your shins. If you're punching them, your knuckles will bruise. Learning is trial and error, hurting yourself to come back stronger. Sooner or later you'll become exactly what you sought all along.

The martial arts bring people back to center. It doesn't matter what brought you to class—whether you needed to expend some energy, were bullied in grade school, or just wanted to learn a new skill. Whatever trauma you've gone through can be fought with the hands. If someone's been bullied and they learn the mechanics to defend themselves, they may never use them to break a bully's nose, but they'll gain the security that was lacking in the first place and was the root of all their fears. And if they end up having to fight, they're prepared.

We spend so much of our time in turmoil. The body's confused because it doesn't get enough activity. The head is confused because it can't let out stress. Your brain and body don't like to argue because it's counterproductive. You'll never get anything done. You have to use both body and mind to be successful. You have to exercise that connection, and running on the treadmill or playing a game of chess isn't enough. You have to strengthen that bond and flex the connection. Martial arts is all about training that focus so you can access it on command.

Ultimately there's nothing better in the world of fitness to humble you than the martial arts. There are so many things to learn that you'll find unlimited potential for improvement. If growth is your goal, welcome. You've come to the right place.

THE VIKING NINJA SIGIL

People constantly ask me about the meaning of the Viking Ninja sigil depicted on the cover of this book. I didn't simply want a logo that looked good to represent the system. I wanted one that carried power in its own right. I like the word sigil because it's what the symbols carved or painted onto shields and flags in the middle ages were called. They said something important about the values and beliefs of whoever bore them.

There isn't an element of the sigil that doesn't have purpose. Like other symbols, without you or me it's nothing but a collection of ink and lines. There's nothing magical about it, rather the power it has comes from what we give it and in turn derive from it. When I see the sigil I'm reminded of how far I've come with this system, as well as of what I have left to give. It's also a source of motivation, as it contains a microcosm of all Viking Ninja's philosophy.

The heavy maces, which represent strength, are the most obvious piece of the image, as they expand beyond everything else with an X that draws the eyes. It's like a target. They sit at that angle for a number of reasons, the most basic being that the head is the heaviest part of the mace.

That position—when held behind your back—is the most powerful you'll ever find. It's a landmark from the steel mace 360 and occurs right before you bring the mace overhead for a crushing blow.

There are two sides to the maces. They're not just for delivering brutal force. Remember, the goal of your training, particularly with weapons and the martial arts, is not to do harm. Viking Ninja is about coming together rather than separating. Thus the cross represents defense. It's protection. When you hold a mace out in front of you, one hand beneath the head and the other at the base of the handle, it's going to withstand every strike that comes your way. We train to stand up for what's right, and the mace is the perfect tool to represent that.

A third idea contained in the maces is brotherhood. There are two of them for a reason. We're not alone: we work united. Viking Ninja isn't about trying to do everything on your own. We thrive off of community, whether that means pushing one other to achieve greatness, working together for the same, or watching each others' backs in times of trouble. When I see those crossed maces I see an impenetrable barrier that nothing can pass. It inspires me to consider my brothers and sisters before myself, and to remember why I do what I do. Viking Ninja isn't about me, but everyone else that's a part of my life and this community.

As with the maces, the shield represents numerous things, though the most important is protection. It protects the meaning of the sigil itself. It implies that our philosophy is safe, that it will never be taken from us. It protects our purpose—strength, understanding, education, and philosophy. It reminds us that though we should always keep an open mind, what we hold dear must be safeguarded. It's easy to forget the old when something bright, shiny, and new enters the picture.

This shield helped my ancestors conquer the North, and they depended on one another to protect and guard each other when they were in danger. The moment you let your shield down and drop the philosophy is the moment you not only open yourself up to harm, but you let down your brothers as well, the people you're responsible for protecting. The Vikings didn't use their shields to protect themselves alone. They weren't selfish. Remember, honor was key to their culture and way of life. The shield protects us from anything that seeks to destroy us, whether in mind, body, or spirit.

The runes say, "Live through your Warrior Spirit and honor your dedication." Those are the most important words in all of Viking Ninja because they provide a succinct roadmap for how to live your life. The Warrior Spirit represents truth, honesty, passion—all the deepest parts of yourself, which for many of us will take a lot of time to uncover. Once we've accessed the Warrior Spirit we have to honor it by respecting ourselves and not allowing ego or destructive impulses to take over.

I also like to imagine the shield as the world. The runes speak to everyone that's part of the community and everyone standing outside it—everyone behind the shield and everyone before it. The maces stick out because our strength is endless. The world can't contain it. And in turn the runes are guarded by Jörmungandr, the Midgard Serpent. In Norse mythology, Odin throws a serpent into the sea that grows so enormous it circles the world and bites onto its own tail.

The legends say that if Jörmungandr ever releases his tail, Ragnarök—the end of the world—will begin. The Midgard Serpent was constantly depicted on ships, leading the way for Vikings. It can't let go, because then the shield crumbles, the world falls apart. All of the philosophy evaporates and Viking Ninja dies. Yet that will never happen. How do you keep the serpent alive? Passion. Your passion for life and growth have to protect the meaning in your heart.

Jörmungandr represents your Warrior Spirit. It's constantly driving to improve itself and cut away the weak by eating the old, eating history, eating what once served it but can now be left behind in the past. The Viking Ninja way is to discard what doesn't help you and to bring in anything that makes you stronger. We aim to break the system and create new rules, a new way of life that will serve us better than the way of yesterday.

The circle is the world and Jörmungandr gives it motion. The world is always turning. It's infinite and never ends. There's always opportunity for growth, and the limits of yesterday are meant to be broken. If you make a mistake, there's room for improvement and to rectify it. The Warrior Spirit is always active. It never sleeps, just like the twenty-four hour Viking and Ninja. One operates by day and one by night, but together they never stop.

Ultimately the sigil represents the passion you need to conquer yourself and become what you've always wanted to be. Having that image to remind yourself of what you want in life is invaluable to success. I'm surrounded by it everywhere I look because Viking Ninja is such a huge part of how I spend my days. It serves as a constant push in every direction.

The colors I chose in the design were not random. Color brings meaning. Can you imagine living in a world of nothing but gray? The sigil is white, black, and red. Red symbolizes blood—your blood, and that you'd spill it for what you believe in. You have to be content with the knowledge that you will bleed to achieve your goals. Everyone has to bleed in battle. Everything you do comes from within. It's in your veins. If you're unwilling to fight for what you believe in, why live in the first place? Go back to your sofa. The happiest, most satisfied people I know are the ones who get up every morning with a purpose, and if you'd let go of that so easily then it was never meant for you in the first place. You've been fooling yourself.

The sigil isn't all positive. It's also a reminder of what not to do. Erik the Red was the most vicious Viking of all time. He ravaged lands, raped women, murdered children. All that destruction and evil led to a short life. It was brutal and hard. Yet what if he'd taken that intensity and put his efforts toward something good? You have to access that same vigor and enact positive change on the world.

We all bleed red, but we also bring black to life. You utilize the black—Ninja—to be content in the dark. You have to be comfortable with the unknown. In the dark you have other senses to rely upon, like touch and sound, yet your instincts have to be on point. It's also the reminder that sometimes we must take our dark, raw energy and put it to use. You have to be resolute, because we all have cancer in our lives that has to be cut away, whether it's the junk food that's poisoning you or the "friends" you hold onto out of fear of loneliness even though all they do is tear you down.

Like the Yin Yang, the sigil is black and white. Ninjas have a little bit of white in their circle to keep them balanced, where as Vikings have black in theirs. Vikings fought during the day, but as you see in the Yin Yang, there's a little dark. They create darkness in light, and the ninjas make light in darkness. It's just enough to balance each other out. Balance is of the utmost importance in all endeavors.

The Ninja aspect isn't as obvious within the sigil as the

Viking. The maces are primary, as is the shield. Yet before you can approach a steel mace or any other weapon, you need the body to operate it. That's where Ninja comes in. *You* are the person in the sigil—you're just not pictured. You're the ninja. You're the Viking. It's your responsibility to change the world and live up to the destiny before you.

IMMORTALITY

Immortality is a major part of Viking Ninja, but with such a huge concept comes a whole variety of possible meanings. If we constantly exceed our limits, where does that take us? Regardless of whether perfection is possible, we're constantly moving in that direction. And somewhere on the spectrum lies immortality.

We aim to defy time as it eats us away. We all have to watch ourselves age, but the process can be slowed down, and in certain cases it even appears to reverse itself. Some people certainly get old faster than others. Yet what's less apparent—and simply because we can't see it—is that the mind and spirit undergo the same process.

As we age our memory fades, our thinking slows, the crispness with which we engage and perceive the world begins to soften. The spirit, too, grows tired. Life's trivialities begin to mount and we grow weary. We lose whatever vigor we once had and instead turn to gelatinous remnants of what we were.

Our mission isn't just about living longer. Who wants that kind of immortality? It's sad, but most of the elderly people I know are just counting the days. How many of them are filled with regret? Only a few seem utterly content with how they lived their lives. If you want to be happy, especially as time passes, you have to conduct yourself in a way that's in accordance with your views and beliefs. We're focused on finding that path and walking it. If you fall off, we're going to pull you back.

I like to think of immortality not just in the sense of length, but in density. You want your life to be rich with experience, so saturated with fascination and novelty that every day is a gem worth holding onto. That's what I mean by dense immortality, and it's what we're seeking—the physical strength, the spiritual vitality, the mentor rigor to fuel that sort of life.

This is something you get to take with you on your journey. You never leave what you did at the gym in the locker room, or what you learned at the library in the stacks of books. Every minute you live with discipline is a minute you win the war, and those victories mount up.

As with anything else in Viking Ninja, it's a self-fueling cycle. Living life with density creates a level of expectation for the future. You're going to expect hard days. Grinding days. Yet you know how they'll make you feel afterward, and you'll be prepared for anything.

You may hate the heavy days. Maybe you hate the light days. It might be you hate the nights you have to spend at the office. But either way you've done them before, you've been there, you've conquered and emerged knowing what victory felt like. And you're going to keep doing it and the gains will continue to mount.

Remember that at our core we're a fitness system, and there are so many ways to immortalize the body. The type of movement we teach will improve your circulation, which everyone needs. I don't care who you are, you need a strong heart. Though most of us think of exercise as only conditioning our muscles, training is just as much about the mind. Viking Ninja challenges the nervous system to keep the body hot-wired from center to its most distal appendages, ensuring that ever more muscle fibers are being recruited to constantly improve your economy of movement.

There's nothing more complex than us. Molecules, atoms, quantum physics? They're peanuts compared to the body, since there are billions and trillions and quadrillions of them inside each and every one of us. Their interactions make them even more complicated than when studying them in isolation.

The body is filled with math and science, and yet it's also the most intuitive piece of equipment we have. A baby can use it, though it takes some time to learn. Still, the body has to be treated as a precious commodity, because we only get one, and all those physics can be mishandled. Apply your knowledge carefully, and take things slowly. If you don't understand something, don't rush through it. That's how we break our hardware, and this isn't a race against anyone or anything but time. It's hard to cheat time, but it can be done. That's what we're searching for, and it takes caution. Don't value speed so much as fluidity. What you want is to be a well-oiled machine, not one that goes all out and burns up the moment it leaves the atmosphere.

Fortify all those little things you need for immortality. Your body has to be able to run smoothly for a long time without huffing and puffing as it begs for the air and nutrients you can't provide since you've neglected to take care of yourself for so long. We stress volume to ensure that all these principles are thoroughly engrained in your mind and body. Learn to treat and maintain yourself like a NASCAR mechanic.

The steel mace is a key tool for achieving immortality. One of the first things to go as we get older is our hands. We lose the connection between mind and body, and the most finite, intricate movements fade first. Old people shake at the hands because their nervous systems are on out-of-control autopilot. If you do a hundred steel mace 360s on each side your hands are going to shake, but that's not weakness, it's stimulation. And that stimulation is going to keep those hands alive for the long haul.

It all starts with your mind. The head has to be strong before the rest. It's going to pull your body along with it. If your mind isn't strong, your body won't want to exert itself when you attempt to exceed your limits. The body doesn't want to be in debt. The body is inherently lazy. Without a mind it will just lie there. That's what comatose patients do, after all. The mind has to provide it with life. Immortality doesn't start in the gym, with what you eat, or how big your biceps are. As immortality applies to the human condition, to life, it all begins in the mind.

You have to look at mental weakness like a disease to be purged in order for survival. Disease is anything you're not comfortable with, any qualities you possess that you don't believe in, that have become part of you despite your best intentions. Laziness, sugar addiction, alcoholism, all of those things are the type of disease I'm talking about here.

You can be strong in so many aspects of life, and yet have one weak point that will always bring you down. That's why the myth of Achilles and his heel is so important for us. We need to find our heels and shore them up. They can be physical or mental.

You can't let life take advantage of your weak spots and play you like a game. You have to be able to untangle your emotions, which means looking them right in the eye. So many of us have problems that in actuality couldn't be more minor, yet as soon as they come around we dig our heads in the ground like ostriches.

Still, immortality isn't just about you. It's not about lifespan or how engaged you are in your daily activities. Immortality is about becoming legendary, and everyone has that potential. You may not become Hercules, but you can at least set a path for your friends, your children, whoever it is. Being immortal means living on through the minds of others to impact the world. The teachings of Viking Ninja aim to bring out that quality in you, and everybody else who takes part. This is because of brotherhood, and also the importance of social awareness and contribution, of sharing what you have with people who have less.

Viking Ninja is a concept that means nothing without the people who believe in it. I may be its founder, but I can't be everywhere at once. I can't be you, and you can't be me. I can only be in so many places, so many gyms, so many late night conversations discussing the meaning of life. It's up to everyone that's part of this community to be a fountain of knowledge, of inspiration and advice, for the people whose lives they touch. Each one of us can be a source of greatness for the world, a well from which others can drink and grow strong. Everyone can become the hometown hero, a legend in their neck of the woods, a legend for their family and descendants.

This role can be squandered or even wholly counterproductive if you aren't responsible. You must live up to your position from an angle of positivity, not negativity. Don't be like Genghis Khan, who conquered the world but left fear and hate everywhere he went. Be a Gandhi or Mother Theresa, spreading love and hope. Be a Bruce Lee, the legend who made me who I am today, freeing people's minds through their bodies.

The ultimate level of immortality in Viking Ninja is attaining a black belt, which means you're constantly exceeding levels. And when you constantly improve, it becomes a lifestyle—one in which every day you're a better, stronger, livelier person than you were the day before.

That's the opposite of normal. This generation is lazy. Weak. And if you're an immortal? Then they drop around you like flies. Compared to the average person, you really are a god walking among mortals. You're growing stronger and smarter with your body in a world that's dumb. It's filled with sheep so reliant on technology they don't know how to use their muscles. The most bleeding-edge equipment on the planet is the human body, and in particular the brain. If you have that in check, then you're astronomically more advanced than anyone else around you. Most people don't know how to control it, and they use technology as a crutch. Their car gets them to the corner store, the microwave cooks their TV dinners that they buy there, and Red Box DVDs fill their empty minds.

Don't head in that direction. Drop the electric scooter and video games. Pick up a steel mace. Get some clubs. Kettlebells. That's how you optimize and reach immortality. When you utilize your body as it's designed to be used rather than relying on outside support, you'll finally shape it into the life machine it's meant to be. Learn to harness your strength. That's the math. That's the science. Use it and achieve immortality.

VIKING NINJA CHAKRA

The Viking Ninja Chakra is the combination of the Valknut, Yin Yang, and Vegvisir Compass. As the element of mind, the Valknut sits in the head. As the element of balance, and in particular of the body, the Yin Yang sits at the core in your abdomen. And as the uniting passion, purpose, and path, the Vegvisir Compass sits in the center of your sternum over your heart, connecting the two and forming a trinity.

The three symbols complete you as a Viking Ninja. If you've managed to find and optimize them, you've unlocked your Warrior Spirit and nothing can defeat you. Though it's a complicated task, the way to acquire and activate the Viking Ninja Chakra is to kill your ego and constantly challenge your discipline.

Possessing the trinity makes you far stronger than the average person, though that doesn't make it a competition. You shouldn't be competing with other people, only yourself. If life beats you down before you can beat life—which means owning yourself and everything you do—then your being here on earth has no purpose. You haven't found a direction.

The Chakra enables you to walk that path. Regardless of whether or not you see any merit in using the symbols I've put forth and that are fundamental to the system, if you have ambition you will likely agree that the keys to fulfillment are balance in mind, body, and spirit as you seek to reach your goals. The Viking Ninja Chakra is just a set of values and checkmarks to help you realize and visualize that process.

It all starts with the mind-bind in the Valknut and the three triangular concepts that compose it, interlocking and intertwining. They don't know how to unify on their own, because the mind is chaotic when left to its own devices. In order to find that solid trinity you need to access the Yin Yang. As long as your center is balanced, your mind will stay balanced. You can read into that whatever you want, but one way I find this in practice is by keeping myself centered through fitness. Training calms the mind and allows me to collect my thoughts. A spastic, unruly body filled with energy struggling to be let out will find itself mirrored in disordered thinking.

The final part is the Vegvisir Compass, which you can only access once you've found your Yin Yang and Valknut. Everyone has all three symbols, yet they're buried under countless layers of aimlessness. The Vegvisir Compass waits in your heart. Once you've reached it you'll have your Warrior Spirit, and with it the Viking Ninja Chakra is complete.

Then you start to reap the benefits that come from understanding your goal and why you're living life the way you do. Everybody and everything has a purpose. They're all different, and yet they boil down to the same difference. It's about winning life, and the only way you do that is by engaging the Chakra to conquer yourself mentally, physically, and spiritually.

Viking Ninja Elements

What's a life with a body and mind but no spirit? You're essentially a robot. A body and spirit but no mind? You're a monkey. No body? How can you engage with the world and express yourself to the fullest? In order to stay disciplined in practice you have to use the Chakra to ensure that you're properly aligned in all facets of your being to follow your path. No matter where you go, since you have the Vegvisir Compass, you'll never be lost. You're going to succeed.

What does the Vegvisir Compass really represent? It may seem like an afterthought to the Chakra, less a crowning piece than something you receive once you've done the real work with the Valknut and the Yin Yang. It's the S on your chest if you're Superman, the bat if you're Batman, the spider if you're Spiderman. It shows that you have purpose, that you're there to serve and you have the powers and attributes to back you up. You're untouchable, invincible, unbreakable, and destined to win. The superhero is always victorious because their heart is in the right place. Once you have the Viking Ninja Chakra in order you're on the path, but you have to continue respecting it because it's a privilege, not a right. You earned it, and you have to keep on earning it if you want to maintain your super powers.

It's not enough to keep the Chakra in mind when you're training. That may work for some things, like sustaining focus or remembering the sequence of movements you're going to perform, but the Chakra isn't only about the mind. It's body and spirit as well. You have to apply the Chakra in everything you do by being a single point of intention, unifying the disparate parts of your being through action.

What is your purpose when training? Where's it taking you? Or are you taking the training somewhere? Once you've challenged yourself and peered around the corner of the next level you get addicted to the possibility of growth. You have to keep applying the Viking Ninja Chakra to continually exceed your limitations. If you want to skip dimensions and visit another world, then be prepared to use every last ounce of energy you have. Bring your Chakra, and don't forget the Vegvisir Compass. It will allow you to take what you learn in that next dimension and then find your way back to ours so that you can implement it into your lifestyle and change the world.

Though Viking Ninja is primarily a fitness system, the Chakra isn't only for the gym. You carry it with you everywhere. It's a training concept that applies to life. When you bring the Chakra home it helps you burn through all challenges. Stress makes you unbalanced, and the next thing to go is your mind. Stress will mess you up worse than the most terrible physical calamity. You'll be vomiting, inflamed, incapable of even getting out of bed. Use the Chakra to destroy it before it reaches you.

The Vegvisir Compass doesn't reward you for panic. If a crew of Vikings take over a ship and then the captain loses control, what was the point? They're not going anywhere, and even if they do make landfall, they'll be defeated. They'll probably crash on rocks far before they reach the shore, regardless. After you lose the compass you have no idea what you're doing, and if you're responsible for other people or tasks, then they go to hell and stress just continues to mount. It's one huge avalanche. Like the ship in chaotic water, your mind and body become unbound in a storm of upheaval.

How do you calm that storm? It's no simple charge, but the Viking Ninja Chakra works like anti-rotation, counter-rotation, and purposeful rotation in steel mace training. It's going to help you stay centered even when internal forces seek to send you out of alignment. When forces outside your control like a storm at sea try to blow you away, you hunker down, engage your Warrior Spirit, and withstand the wind by not bending or breaking no matter what gets thrown at you. And when you're ready, you take your purpose and use that strength to fuel you and your crew out of the mess.

The Chakra is complete once you have the three elements in line, and they don't all come at once. You can have only the Yin Yang or only the Valknut, but not only the Vegvisir Compass. Still, once you have both the Yin Yang and the Valknut, you likely have the Vegvisir Compass. You can be perfectly balanced in body but not have your mind right. You can also be extremely composed but lack a strong body. Once you kill your ego and engage your discipline it's only a matter of time before you find the proper alignment to embark upon your journey.

If you're at sea and you get lost, it's your responsibility. It's also on you if you're responsible for people aboard the ship, or if you sabotage somebody else's journey. If you're on a championship team and you get distracted by something outside the game and you cost the team victory, it's nobody's fault but yours. You have to own your Chakra. Your ego must be killed. Your discipline must be challenged. The Valknut and Yin Yang must be stable to hold up the Vegvisir Compass and unite the trinity.

At the end of the day it comes back to Total Human Optimization—Onnit and Viking Ninja just have different ways of describing it. The Vegvisir Compass points you in the direction of Total Human Optimization and the Chakra contains all the elements that in the end will take you there. The Vegvisir Compass doesn't operate by itself. Without a balanced mind and body you're a liability, not only to yourself, but to whoever's ship you're on, whether that's Onnit, Viking Ninja, or any other community. There are no ifs, ands, or buts about it.

BELTING SYSTEM

This chapter is about the structure of Viking Ninja's educational arm, but more generally addresses meritocracy and our attitudes toward mastery and self-responsibility. What I advocate with Viking Ninja is a belting system, which I distinguish from the more typical level system. These are just the names that I'm giving the two for the purpose of making it easier to describe them, as they don't have generally agreed upon terms in our day-to-day language since we rarely talk about them.

The distinguishing factor between the systems is arbitrariness. A level system is arbitrary and doesn't recognize the different needs and abilities of individuals. A coach operating under this philosophy might say, "The next level to the squat is this. It's set in stone, so don't question me." On the other hand, I believe the "next level" to a squat is distinct in every situation. Progressions and regressions apply to individual people with unique bodies and mechanics, and they translate differently to each person's situation and goals.

A level system follows the ego and progresses to advanced work without purpose. There's no reasoning to it. If a coach tells you to squat hop for two straight minutes, they clearly don't understand how to train and develop a skill set. They've hit a wall. All they know is to break someone down and hurt them. That's what they call mastery, and it's irresponsible. At the end of the day the body grows confused and you don't reap any rewards.

A belting system revolves around philosophy. There's nothing arbitrary about it. If you earn your stripes through performance, your body is speaking the proper language and learning the technique.

In a level system, the currency is time, money, or sweat, not understanding. It's like Warcraft players who skip the effort by paying to level up versus the people who grind through the game to gain experience. The first gamer loses out on all the benefits, all the richness of life just to display a number, whereas the latter gets to enjoy the journey.

Show your worth, not how much you're worth. Constantly remind yourself why you're doing what you're doing. You can't ever lose sight of that, or else you end up going through the motions, treading water and not moving forward. It's my responsibility as a coach to do the same. If people don't know why I'm having them do something, they'll half-ass it, expecting to move along like it's a time-based level system. But that's not what I want. You don't get an A for showing up.

In Viking Ninja, any certification is pass or no-pass. It's a four-level belting system. Each belt means something else, and different people will pass into them for different reasons. You don't get a white belt—the first belt—just for showing up. That's the opposite of what we stand for. You have to study, practice, and pass a test. We aren't handing out free cookies. This is hard, serious work, and you have to prove yourself if you want to gain rank.

Now, the white belt is not complex. It begins with the foundations of the system. Just because it's merit-based doesn't mean I'm trying to kill people with difficult work. I want success. First we work with bodyweight because it's central to all movement, especially work with weapons and tools.

You'll learn to accelerate and decelerate through different positions. After bodyweight we transition to the steel mace, which is the cornerstone of all Viking Ninja training. Whereas a lot of the bodyweight movements will be linear, the steel mace is inherently prone to rotation. That doesn't mean we're getting overly complex, as you still have to remain disciplined. Safety is always a primary concern in physical training. Here we learn about anti-rotation, which breeds both awareness and control. You have to be the master of the mace if you wield it.

The belting system requires being responsible with progression and regression. In school they move everybody up at the same pace regardless of performance. With Viking Ninja it's about what you do and how you do it, not showing up. Everybody moves at a different pace, but there's nothing wrong with that. We're all unique, with different aptitudes in different areas. At school if you get a D- you pass, and I say no to that. There are no D- Viking Ninja black belts. I won't have it.

The while belt helps you understand our foundation, both in movement and philosophy. That means bodyweight, the steel mace, and applying yourself toward killing the ego and challenging your discipline. It's designed to work you all over—body, mind, and spirit.

The blue belt is more advanced. Here we take the basics and apply more complexity. The third belt is the red belt. To reach this level you have to understand and demonstrate movement to the highest degree of difficulty. Reaching the final belt, the black belt, is different from the rest. Rather than learning more material, it's about proving your mastery.

With the belting system also comes accountability. Let's

say you pass the white belt test. You work hard, do all the preparation, and then after a year you hit the blue belt. Yet then you get lazy. You stop training and rest on your laurels. Sorry, that just won't cut it. This is an honor, a responsibility, and definitely not a right. You better believe you're gonna get knocked back to white belt. You proved you weren't ready. You're not honoring your dedication. That's not at all what Viking Ninja is about.

The path is always to the black belt. Why get a blue belt and then grow lazy? The goal is always black. You're here to exceed your limitations and constantly grow, right? This isn't just about fun. You're on the hunt, and the hunt has no end. It doesn't end at the black belt, either. To have reached that level means you understand the importance of growth. You don't need me dangling a carrot in from of you anymore. You're going to constantly improve on your own. There is no end to this journey.

You must have an empty cup to participate in the Viking Ninja belting system, but we aren't close-minded and dogmatic like some schools. Certainly we have our own rules, but we're not going to kick you out if you train somewhere else.

But just because we're open-minded doesn't mean you can do anything you want. If you're in some weirdo suicide-cult, maybe Viking Ninja isn't the place for you. Don't do things that make people uncomfortable. Don't be someone you're not. Express yourself, but be honest. Nothing's off limits. Still, you may learn things through Viking Ninja that turn you off to other systems.

There are rewards for each belt, and people who fail can always retest. It will require more work, though. Yet whose fault is that? You should have prepped harder and done more work in the beginning. We warned you. We're warning you right now. Be ready. This is no joke. I design these tests so that people can be proud of their accomplishments when it's all said and done. This is meant to be a revelatory experience, not something you forget about the next day.

The belting system gives us goals and structure, but we all have to find our own path. We're too scared to face our problems. People ignore them because they're frightening. They sweep them under the rug and move on to the next thing. That's not how it should be. That's how you amass problems, and pretty soon you're weighed down and there's nowhere left to go. Then you're living a lie and putting on a fake smile, even though whenever you're alone you're crying and stressed and can't get anything done. You're a ship that's slowly sinking.

That's the course of more and more lives these days. We lack the strength to confront our problems and move forward. That's what I'm fighting against. Everything we do in the gym is preparation for life, not just fitness. We're strengthening our discipline to such a degree that there isn't a thing that can stop us.

BROTHERHOOD

Without community, we're lost. But it can mean so many things at different times and places that it's tough to discuss coherently. What does brotherhood mean at war? What does it mean in the kitchen of a high class restaurant? What does it mean when serving soup at a homeless shelter?

At the center of the word is "brother." That's family. There's love in it. Kinship. Brotherhood means treating people as if they're your own flesh and blood, as if they're part of you. That's what unites the soldiers, the chefs, the people who live indoors and out. Brotherhood is about treating others like family.

It's easy to hate, to be mean, to bully. It's an unfortunate fact of life that it's natural. Chimpanzees tear each other apart. Ants battle with neighboring colonies. As advanced as we may think we are, we still have wars going on all over the world and crime occurring on every city block. It requires a higher order of humanity, another level of discipline and emotional capacity, to take your love, your energy, and share it with people around you.

We naturally gravitate toward those whose beliefs and values resonate with ours. They're who we form strong bonds with and in time call brothers and sisters. As these bonds strengthen, we grow comfortable. We feel safe. You can call on those people for help and guidance whenever you need it, and that's invaluable. There are times when we all need support. Being lonely is the worst feeling of all. It's hopeless. It's dread. It's what leads to depression and stagnation. It prevents progress.

The worst betrayal is when brotherhood gets faked. That's why all throughout history and mythology it's the liars and traitors who get punished worst. Think of Judas and Brutus. There's a reason Satan chews on them for eternity in Dante's Inferno. But even to a lesser extent, we plaster brotherhood on bonds that are far weaker and mean nothing of the sort. Sometimes you're just part of a team or unit, or you're working with someone on the same project, but that doesn't mean you're brothers.

If your coworker a few doors down dies, are you going to send his children to college? Probably not, yet if that was your bunkmate at war, you bet your ass you'd do everything you could to provide for their family. Teams break up all the time. Maybe your coworker gets a promotion and you never see him again.

But brotherhood is strong. There's no breaking up. If they wrong you, you forgive them. You never abandon your brothers. If you ever find people in your life like that, you have to hold onto those relationships like your life depends on it, because it just might. If you're in a dark place, they can help.

Brotherhood is about love. You never abandon someone you love. "Abandon" is the word I hate most in the English language, because I was abandoned as a kid. My dad was never around. My mother raised my brother and I, and family is all you have. Brotherhood is everything. *Everything.* You don't want to be lonely. I can't imagine the pain of growing old and watching my loved ones die. That's one reason Viking Ninja is so important to me. I want to prolong everyone's life so that people can stay around happier and healthier, and not only for themselves, but for those around them who care.

Brotherhood and Viking Ninja are inseparable. We take care of each other. We're far stronger together than we are separate. I know it's cliche, but you've seen the movie 300. Brotherhood is more than just holding up a shield to guard your friend's back. It's about caring and being thoughtful,.

In Viking Ninja we're all connected by the same mission—self-improvement. We aim to live through the Warrior Spirit and honor our dedication. Our goals have a similar flavor, but they're still all different. There are lawyers, physicians, athletes, and though our objectives may take different appearances, they all require identical discipline, dedication, and commitment—everything contained by the Valknut, Yin Yang, and Vegvisir Compass.

Rather than just doing our own thing and living in our own little bubbles, we think about one another and how to offer support. We push each other harder in the gym so that we can work better outside it. We back each other's endeavors in every way we can, whether that's sports-related or otherwise. If you're putting on a comedy show, I'm gonna be there. If you need me to test out a new recipe at your restaurant, I'm definitely going to be there.

Brotherhood is a self-fueling entity. Every minute you spend with someone you care about results in a stronger bond and deeper unity. Brotherhood isn't about seeing someone once and then calling them three months later. It's a daily thing where you're truly invested in that other person and they're invested in you. Brotherhood means nagging and annoying the hell out of someone if they need to get something done but are ignoring it. You're there to make them better and give them that extra nudge, and in the end they're going to appreciate it and do the same for you.

Brotherhood is continuous communication. We're here to keep each other accountable for the goals we set. The brotherhood, as they say, is only as strong as its weakest link. If you're in a military unit, you don't want a slacker in your squad. You want everyone to be stronger, better, and faster than you are so that if you're in a pinch you're surrounded by people that can be counted on.

Keep the friends who expect you to be disciplined, dedicated, and positive. Those are good friends. Those are the people you want in your life. The people who drag you down, throw them in the dumpster and never look back. If you're that kind of person and aren't committed to changing, then put down this book. You're not right for our community. Sorry.

If you're fake, if you only consider yourself, if you're trying to extract every bit of wealth you can from other people, then you're a slave to your ego. You're selfish and distracted from execution, from exceeding your limits. You're not honoring the beauty and commitment of what brotherhood is all about.

The Viking Ninja way is to keep your word. When I tell someone I'm going to do something, I'm going to help them out, I follow through with it. But it's not true brotherhood if they expect you to do all the heavy lifting. They have to get out and help push the wagon, too. Holding your hand out for freebies goes against everything I've just described. We're talking about brotherhood, not theft.

Where's the brother in you that's going to help me push when my car breaks down? That's when you know who your real friends are. I hold my people accountable for that sort of stuff. It's the truest judge of character there is. People will jump on your wagon when you're successful and living in the limelight, but where do they go when things aren't so flush anymore? The real friends help push your car out of the ditch. They don't run off when nobody's looking.

People will ask you for money, they'll ask you to do stuff for free. You have to prove your worth before someone lets you into their circle. Don't ask for handouts. Give before you take. That's how you make meaningful relationships and earn trust. If you start taking without giving, then you harm the brotherhood. And if you have no choice but to take, then you better give back ten times more once you have the capacity.

Brothers make sacrifices. That's how you show your love. Yet sacrifices aren't a negative thing. It's about protection. We give up for the whole. A single mother gives up everything—social time, friendships, freedom—to protect her family. Nobody has more dedication or Warrior Spirit than she does. If everybody in a brotherhood acted with that same honor and selflessness, the community would be indestructible. Everyone needs to be a leader. Everyone needs to be dedicated, to make sacrifices. It becomes effortless. And if you're still struggling, your brothers will help you out. Anything is surmountable when you have a community.

Think of the Vikings, who honored one another to a fault. When they went into battle together, they watched each other's backs. They avenged death. They went to Valhalla together. Regardless of whether or not that's a real place, it's the attitude you have to take. You're in it with your brothers until the end. That's how you push past the hard stuff, how you dig deep in the final minutes to win the championship, to bring your wounded comrade home from battle when you have to carry him ten miles in the blistering heat. If your friend dies at war, you bury him in a place of honor and care for his family, and he'll do the same for you.

The goal in Viking Ninja is to build an environment where nobody feels alone. I want everyone to feel the support of a hundred people who are going through the same thing, who have been there in the past. Whether you want to be a ninja or a barbarian, I want someone who's been there to help you through your transformation.

Brotherhood in Viking Ninja is more than just fitness. It's about living a life you can be proud of, one that's full of love and laughter. Everything in the wild is tough. We have to scramble to survive. It's a dark forest, and we all fight for the light. But we can make our lives sweeter by going through that journey with our hands clasped together. It makes us stronger, and it makes that forest just a little bit safer. If you fall, we'll help you back up. If you succeed, you'll pull us up with you. It's easier to commit toward excellence when you're working with people who want the same thing. It's all about the push and pull.

RECOVERY

Day in and out all we think about is go, go, go. The readily apparent result is that we're worn down. Our bodies are broken, our minds slow and tired, and our spirits lack passion and resolve. It may seem like Viking Ninja is setting you on that same path. After all, killing the ego and challenging your discipline sounds aggressive, or at the very least exhausting.

Yet that's not the case. Recovery is every bit as important as the self-development aspect of the system. Lifting weights and moving strains the body. You leave the gym weaker than when you entered. Strength gains occur when your muscles knit themselves back together, adapting to the stress you put them through so that they can return more efficient and capable. Though the direct connection can't be so easily explained when considering the mind and spirit, the same principles apply. If you never allow your mental faculties time off, they will only grow more weary until they cease to function.

If people consider recovery at all, they typically think it means sleep, which is extremely important—maybe the most important ingredient of all—but far from sufficient to fix all our wear and tear. Yes, your joints and muscles will heal when you rest, but eight hours with your eyes closed isn't enough to rejuvenate the mind.

Life will beat you down. There are times when we have to keep going and push through fatigue, but eventually your spirit will exhaust itself. If the mind and body don't recover they won't perform at a high level and will ultimately sustain lasting damage in the form of physical injury or mental illness.

The more you exert yourself without devoting time to recovery, the less balanced you become. The Yin Yang begins to fade away as your body weakens. The mind-bind tangles once again as you lose peace of mind. No matter how much passion you have, if you rely on it incessantly it will drain. You may have the capacity to burn like a blowtorch, but once the gas is gone no matter how hard you pull the trigger nothing's going to come out. Be a candle with a long, sturdy wick that takes forever to burn.

If we're composed of mind, body, and spirit, we have three elements that need recovery. That's a lot of work, and unfortunately we have limited time. It's rare to see people take time away from exercising to strengthen their bodies with a foam roller, stretching, or some other durability implement, and you never see people sitting at the gym in meditation. As time is such a scarce resource, an ideal recovery practice enables you to nurture all three elements of your being at once.

Thus recovery comes from the center, the Yin Yang, because recovery depends on balance. You can't speed through this process, which we all skew toward because we're inherently impatient. We cut short our sleep. We eat quickly by getting fast food instead of cooking and enjoying wholesome meals. We rarely, if ever, take the time to slow down and live with our thoughts through meditation or some other form of quiet time. This last one, in particular, ends up harming us through our sleep, as once we get in bed our minds race. It's nearly impossible to go from a hundred miles per hour to a full stop in a short period of time.

You can't be headstrong during recovery. If you think you know everything, you're wrong. We all take the same tinpot stretching routine we did in our high school sports program, do it once or twice a week—if that—and think we deserve a medal. The science of recovery is constantly changing as we learn more about the body, and if you don't have the time to constantly read about it, find a coach who does. You should spend as much time in active recovery as you do exerting yourself. And just as the body needs to be presented with novel stimuli to develop strength, we also feed on fresh recovery modalities so that we don't adapt and cease progressing.

If you're burnt out, cast away your ego. Think deeply about where you came short. Figure out what you're doing right. Cut away the bad, keep the good, and make it more efficient. Whenever you're engaged in a recovery practice you need to be conversing with your body. That means not watching TV or picking at your callouses. Listen to your muscles and tendons to find out what they need. We've grown distant from ourselves, and this time constitutes very necessary remedial education.

Vital to recovery is reconnecting with your purpose. If you have no aim, of course you're going to fatigue. If you're running on a hamster wheel with no end in sight, you're going to fry. Constantly remind yourself of the ultimate goal. Recall your plan. How did you get here in the first place?

Keeping this in mind enables you to return back to your roots. If you can't do that, maybe you're somebody new and shouldn't be doing what's exhausting you now. Maybe you lost your Vegvisir along the way and need to re-evaluate the course of your life. I get tired, myself. I work long hours. But I never consider giving up. This is my path and passion, and it keeps me pushing through whatever difficulties come my way.

The first step to any recovery process is dialing down the volume. If you're listening to music and exhausted, you don't turn the amplifier to eleven. You twist it back to get some sleep. We're so disconnected with ourselves that instead of being compassionate and listening to our cries for help, we smother them and continue working insane hours or training at an unsustainable pace. All you have to do is turn the volume down a little bit. Cut back on your hours behind the desk or treadmill. Kill your toxic relationships.

Recovery is about compassion. It's about forgetting the ten million squats you were supposed to do today. It's about accepting that your back is broken instead of punishing yourself for being lazy. Then you take that hour and stretch, sit in the sauna, or lie in a dark room and breathe, all while playing over the days, weeks, and months behind you. That's when you figure out where you went wrong and how to get back on track.

Chances are you're too tense. We all are. You're doing too much. Slow down. Rest. In the end, who cares? Your success will ultimately depend on your discipline, which requires energy to feed on. As soon as you have the body, mind, and spirit aligned, your passion comes to life and you're ready to get back at it with the rekindled fire you need to exceed your limitations.

The specific recovery methodologies of Viking Ninja are too numerous and complex to list here. After all, this is a book about philosophy, not training programs. But in general, recovery starts with the Yin Yang. You have to completely shut off the body. Whether that means sitting down, meditating, or lying in bed, you should have nothing on your mind except for the thoughts that drift naturally in and out of your consciousness. That means no television or podcasts—nothing that's going to take you out of your body.

Challenge your discipline. Close your eyes and find the hurt. Where are you aching? Where are you compensating for weaknesses? Once you've come to understand your body you can ask what it needs and you'll get honest answers. Your inflamed knee will tell you to give it rest, that the ten miles of running you've been doing every day aren't helping anyone, least of all you. This process is all about turning down the volume so you can hear the quietest sounds, the whispers from your joints and muscles that you've droned out.

Once you've lowered the volume you can turn to your mind and ask those same questions. Now we're addressing the Valknut. This is harder, because the body won't lie. If your knee hurts, you're going to feel it. But we lie to ourselves all the time. Kill your ego and whatever's trying to hold back the truth. What's on your mind more than anything else? What insecurities are holding you back in life? How relevant are they to your goals, or are you making mountains out of molehills? Don't waste your energy. Don't get so involved in your emotions that they ruin your life.

The body has to stay calm as you venture through the mind. Have you ever seen a man on fire while he's meditating? That should be your goal. To calm the mind, to listen to it, to find inner peace despite whatever's happening outside. You're killing the ego one step at a time as each truth rings its way through your head. You're sacrificing yourself to live through your Warrior Spirit. You're untouchable, unbreakable, impenetrable. This is how you should feel after every recovery session: as if you're ready to take on the world.

FLOW (MINDFUL MECHANICS)

If you've made it this far, you've noticed a trend: words, ideas, symbols, they can all have a wide variety of interpretations. Flow is no exception. It has technical meanings in the science world, conventional applications in day-to-day conversation, and field-specific connotations in fitness.

I think of flow as a visual, auditory, or performed expression of artistic intention. Movement in Viking Ninja is not only about rigidly following the rules and becoming another clone. That being said, following rules is the first step, as you need to master the basics before you can express yourself well enough to give them your own spin. Once we've achieved that foundational level of proficiency we can begin to explore the artistic side of movement, and that begins with flow.

Unfortunately, the word flow has been murdered in the fitness setting. It's been killed. I do still like to use it with regard to energy and mentality in line with Eastern movement philosophies like Tai Chi. What I originally took flow to mean in the fitness world was taking the movements you knew and linking them together with purpose and mindful engagement to build a series that could be endlessly repeated or otherwise manipulated to create different forms of expression.

In Viking Ninja I now use the term mindful mechanics in place of flow to distinguish it from what other people out there are doing, though I will use them interchangeably in this chapter. You have to utilize the rise and fall of your energy and intention to succeed in movement. If you lose that connection your work becomes mindless, and then you start to dive into something different, something aimless. Aimlessness never leads to progress.

Flow is a signature element of the Onnit Academy system, and at Viking Ninja we embrace it with every tool at the gym—kettlebells, barbells, battle ropes, suspension, steel clubs, the mace, and anything else you can move with. It doesn't necessarily come at the end of a program, but it incorporates all the skills you've acquired up to that point. Flow is where you take what you've learned and make it yours.

Simply put, mindful mechanics means sequencing movements to form a pattern. With the steel mace a basic flow might involve moving from a lap squat to an archer curl to a 360 and then performing those exercises on the other side. Flow itself is not simple, even if the pattern makes it appear that way.

Mindful mechanics is the ultimate form of mastery you can display with your mace, as it combines what you've learned with your control of mind and body. To flow properly is to link everything together—knowledge, ability, purpose—and turn them into seamless expression.

What distinguishes flow from other training modalities is the creativity it requires. Not only is artistry necessary to design a routine, but as everyone articulates flow differently, the execution itself is unique to the mover. Though you can imagine a class of twenty people doing switch squats for an hour with nearly identical form, when constructing a flow you are alone with the mace. It's your responsibility to pick which exercises go together—and why—and to then determine how they should be performed.

This is the self-expressive component of mindful mechanics. Perhaps you're a martial artist whose goal is to learn the tool from a combat perspective. Your flow may include movements like the 360, uppercut, and bayonet strike bound together to form a successive barrage of blows against a single opponent. But what about multiple opponents? Or maybe you have to incorporate defensive moves. The flow is ever-changing with respect to what *you* need from it.

Your expression is seasoned by more than just your interests. Among other concerns, it's affected by your emotional state at any given moment. If you enter the gym full of exuberance because you're expecting a package of steel maces to be delivered later that day, maybe you incorporate dynamic movements and bounce to your flow so that you can get out all your butterflies. If you're expecting a slew of pricy bills, maybe something more somber would be appropriate.

I refer to flow as mindful mechanics to emphasize technique. Many people come to the gym, pick up a mace for the first time, and begin jumping around with it before they've earned that right. At the very least, flowing requires basic knowledge of the tool and how to move fluidly. The first part of fluidity is mental engagement. It may not always be conscious, as when moving you shouldn't be absorbed in every last detail of performing your exercises—that's what you did in your training beforehand—yet you must be aware of your place in the flow. Where are you coming from? Where are you going? You must also remember your purpose.

The same is true of the body. You have to be ready for movement at any time, whether you're finishing an exercise, in transition, or beginning another. But the mace or other tool is the last piece of your attention-puzzle. You must have the ideal tension and positioning for the next rotation ready to fire like a bullet in the chamber. You must be warm so that you can move safely and effectively. The mind is only half of the flow, and though the body may be the more obvious part, many people neglect to prepare it adequately.

Both pieces function together as one. Countless hours spent with the mace condition them to work in unison, but you must also be focused and ready to work. The mind-body connection is integral to giving basic movements purpose. This is the difference between a sequence of split squats performed to sculpt your butt and a pattern meant to express.

The final result is more than movement—it's a mental state distinct from the expression of mindful mechanics. You can reach this form of consciousness when playing music, sports, or simply thinking hard about a problem. To be in a flow state means that you forget everything other than the task at hand, losing yourself in the present. This requires vast experience and inner calm, but also the proper attitude and a passion for your work. Entering a flow state is always the goal, as it results in the deepest sense of satisfaction.

There are many potential positives to mindful mechanics beyond self-expression and attaining a higher mental state. Perhaps most obvious, flow is just another way to exercise and change up the pace. Many people fall off their programs because they become bored. At Viking Ninja we have many tools and endless possibilities to avoid this outcome, though mindful mechanics in itself provides infinite ways to challenge yourself and break a sweat.

Viking Ninja Elements

When designing a flow you must first take into account its purpose. Is this your warm-up, cool-down, or primary focus for the session? Or is it something else? I structure my mindful mechanics with the following concept in mind: don't overwhelm the body, as then you lose control, which is foundational to flow. You also shouldn't ask too little, as to enter the flow state of mind requires challenge and concentration. You want to program exactly what your body can take—no more and no less. Then you can be certain you've put everything into your work and expressed yourself with all that you can. Think of the Yin Yang and optimizing balance.

Mindful mechanics are also an opportunity to manipulate the modes of movement: static, fluid, and dynamic. To truly master your tool, you must have an understanding of all three—how they make you feel, when you want to use them, and how to control the mace under each condition.

Beyond the metaphysical, balance is among the most neglected aspects of conventional strength training. At its most fundamental level, balance is the relationship between our bodies and the earth. Flowing with the mace and battling its offset weight will keep you in touch with your feet and their connection to the ground, refining your stability in all axes.

Maintaining a proper relationship with the ground is only the first part of the equation. The next is keeping the rest of your body in sync throughout the course of your flow. Moving under offset weight, changing levels, and rotation train full-body stability through your ranges. This is of paramount importance especially for athletes, who rarely play their sports in single planes where balance is easiest.

I've found mindful mechanics to be particularly beneficial for posture. Though there are exceptions, with the right cueing most people can change their alignment to at least approximate proper posture. But without constant intention, we will inevitably return to our poor alignment. Flow gives us an opportunity to make good posture second-nature even in the most arduous circumstances.

Once you're comfortable flowing with one implement, you have a new skill set that can be applied elsewhere. Every tool in the gym has its own strengths, weaknesses, and purposes, and you may choose to use different ones depending on your goals. Though each tool requires its own working knowledge before you incorporate it into anything approximating mindful mechanics, the same principles will apply. You will employ your chosen weapon as an expression of identity through unique movement.

You could flow with a pen or a wheelbarrow, and you can put down your tool at any point during your mindful mechanics. For example, after performing a 360, you might drop the mace (providing you are outside or somewhere safe) and sprawl to the ground as if in battle. Then you could pick up the mace and resume your flow. Bodyweight exercises are always a welcome addition to any routine.

The following are pieces of advice I've found particularly useful when teaching mindful mechanics:

Be the Weapon, Do Not Look Like the Weapon

As soon as we pick up a mace, most of us tend to act like a Berserker from a thousand years ago. While it may look frightening in the mirror, you're more a danger to yourself in this state than you are to anyone else. *Be the weapon*, focusing on form and tension, as it is you—not the mace—that must be ready to strike at any moment.

Aim with Your Flow—Do Not Be Aimless

Always have direction. Be mindful of the exercises you're performing, how you're performing them, and why you're performing them. Otherwise you will become complacent and listless. A successful flow is one that has purpose and is executed accordingly. Without intention you may as well put down your mace. It's a tool, not a toy.

Make Hard Look Easy, Make Easy Look Hard

This concept is similar to our saying, "Make light heavy and make heavy light." A simple movement like an overhead press should not look easy. You should have complete tension, your posture should be excellent, and your position should leak no strength. If it looks hard, you're doing it right. On the other hand, when you're performing a complex sequence, as in mindful mechanics, don't stumble about or flail. The series must run smoothly, appearing as if there's no strain in your body.

Engage Your Body Before the Mace

Before you use the mace you must master your body, or at the very least have control over it. After you've picked up a tool, take the time to find your breath, adopt your ready position, and then engage full-body tension as you optimize your alignment. Only once you've owned your center should you begin to work.

Become a Single Point of Focus

When flowing, your body and mind are one. Yet first your body, with all its disparate parts, must find unity. As you practice, learn to connect your hands to your feet to your breath to your gaze to everything in between. The body is meant to work as a unit, and if you move like a marionette you'll never find fluidity.

Mind the Details

Though your goal is intangible, this doesn't change the premise of flow: mindful mechanics. When perfecting your routine you must be conscious of everything your body does. Are you distributing your weight evenly? How well are your hand switches timed? Are you white-knuckling the mace when a relaxed grip would be better? Minding these details will eventually happen subconsciously, but when honing technique it's best to be aware of everything you can absorb.

Remember the Valknut

Recall that the first trinity of the Valknut contains three concepts: *anti-rotation*, *counter-rotation*, and *purposeful rotation*. The second triangle reflects the *mind*, *body*, and lastly *intention*, which links the two. The third trinity holds *weapon*, *trophy*, and *power*. The Valknut and its ideals should always be committed to heart when flowing. This doesn't mean you need to recite them word for word, but only that you honor the Warrior Spirit as you move.

EDUCATION

Education is non-negotiable. It's impossible to become a stronger, smarter, faster, all-around better person without learning. Growth is predicated on taking in fresh material and incorporating it into your being. Our bodies are built of food, but our minds and spirits develop from experience, ideas, relationships, and all manner of intangible nourishment.

When someone asks me if they can be part of Viking Ninja, I don't start teaching them by taking out a steel mace and doing 360s. I begin with philosophy. That they're asking in the first place signals they're ready to engage in something greater than themselves. The mind comes first, and only afterward does the body follow.

The quality of education hinges on your teacher. Books like this one are powerful, but nothing substitutes a living, breathing person. Everyone has had professors who sat at the front of the room and read straight from the text. That's worthless. I hope to lead by example and teach in a meaningful way. That means knowing the student and delivering the material in a manner that resonates with whatever they're going through.

Still, my goal when teaching Viking Ninja is essentially the same for every person, though it takes different forms. I want people to absorb knowledge that will contribute to their overall resilience and adaptability. Though the applications can at times be trivial, mastering yourself has a tremendous impact on your quality of life. Let's say you hate going to the mall. People there drive you nuts, maybe it's the consumerism, who knows. But your girlfriend loves the mall and drags you there on Saturdays. It ruins your day and you become a grump. We need to work on your character, because nothing external to your mind should be able to compromise your experience of life. I want you to enter the mall and come out unfazed. Maybe you're even happier because you know it made your girlfriend's day.

That's obviously a superficial example, yet the same principle applies when your car breaks down or you lose your job. That doesn't mean nothing hurts, but you can't let anything or anyone other than you control your life. Take responsibility for your actions and reactions. That's the goal of this philosophy—teaching you how to live on your own terms without exception.

The gym is our testing ground. If you can learn to grind with every workout, nothing outside the gym will be able to rattle your cage. Fitness becomes training for your mind to handle stress so that when you visit the mall with your girlfriend or your cat dies you can keep it together and emerge stronger on the other side. You develop the capacity to strap in your brain and body with all the harnesses and protection necessary for the ride, no matter how bumpy it is.

As mentioned above, education requires a teacher—and that teacher will often be you. There can be no compromises, and if you take that responsibility half-assed, you're nothing more than a substitute. I'm not throwing substitutes in the gutter, but a substitute teacher has insurmountable disadvantages. She can never be prepared for class because she hasn't been there for the past year developing and implementing the curriculum. You're at sea without a sail or paddle. As soon as that happens, quality goes off with the wind. The boat is stuck at the whims of the ocean.

Still, everybody starts out that way. When you first accept responsibility and decide to own your actions, you begin with a blank slate. And like the substitute teacher, you have to dig in your heels and get to work. Go out and jog. Read one of Bruce Lee's books. Pick up the trash littered around you.

We all learned the basic principles of education in school, even if we were bad students. You know the rules. Stop talking and pay attention. If you miss a rep when exercising, focus and get back to work. Ultimately it comes down to taking responsibility for your outcomes.

If you're incapable of getting from point A to B by yourself, then find someone or something that can help. You're not a toddler anymore with a parent to pick up after everything you do. Eventually you have to take ownership of life. If you disrespect your goals, you'll only end up feeling sorry for yourself later. To hell with feeling sorry for yourself. Bite your tongue and prove yourself. Deep down you know far more than can ever bubble out from the surface in the form of consciousness. Tap into that and become legendary.

There are levels to education. You don't start with calculus. First you have to count. Though there's debate about the way it's structured, grades in school have their place and purpose. It doesn't make sense to teach kids and adults in the same classroom. Viking Ninja is one unified system, yet every individual operates at their own level. Still, the goal is always the same—to master the material, wherever you are, so that you can ascend and continue onward, exceeding your limitations and becoming a new, better person with every breath you take.

The idea of achieving excellence keeps us challenging ourselves. Never grow complacent. So, you think you've mastered the steel mace? Then it's time to pick up nunchucks. Start striking. There's always a new area in which to improve, and you're not living through your Warrior Spirit or honoring your dedication if you grow comfortable with the mediocre.

Education with Viking Ninja isn't just about training your mind and body. It's not about dissecting the Valknut or perfecting the next progression in your bo staff practice. It's about becoming stronger in life. If darkness falls over you, turn to the light. If there's too much light, find darkness. We're training for balance, because otherwise your mind-bind goes to hell.

You have to meet challenges with an equal but opposite force. Learn to neutralize whatever tries to squash you. If you come home from work and your spouse is shouting because you forgot to take out the trash, meet him or her with kindness and understanding. Maybe they had a terrible day. Fighting that same energy with violence and anger won't solve anything. It's like Bruce Lee said: be water, adapting to whatever situation you find yourself in.

Follow the path set forth by your Vegvisir Compass. If you have to go to war, then go—your mind-bind will be so strong you can't fail. If you're in a fight, take the knowledge you've gained from your bodyweight training and striking, and in turn educate whoever challenged you. Take what you've learned and become the teacher. Engage the darkness, which in this case is your raw power, but because you're balanced, you use your light, your empathy and discipline, to remain responsible. Your goal isn't to hurt anyone, it's to diffuse the situation.

After a fight you pick up your opponent and ask if he's okay. Viking Ninja is about ending fights before they begin, or at the very least ending them quickly and initiating peace talks. Education revolves around developing your character just as much as it does strengthening your body or pouring facts into your brain. On the cover of this book it says, "Kill your ego, challenge your discipline," not, "Memorize the periodic table of elements," or, "Master the splits." The mind needs to be developed first. Without the ground, what use are feet?

Ultimately education comes down to bettering yourself. We want to live fulfilling lives for ourselves and the people around us that we love and care about. Education finds us many forms, but its value is determined by how it directly impacts that purpose. Some people sit in the dark corners of libraries amassing knowledge they'll never need because they're afraid of what's out there in the real world. They escape from it by over-preparing. Others do the same thing at the gym.

Engage your Viking Ninja Chakra to find a path. From there determine what you need to learn if you hope to walk it. Then decide how to acquire that knowledge. Once you've absorbed it, take the final step: implementation.

If your goal is to be a master mover, textbooks will only get you so far. Find the best teachers in the world and allow them to show you their systems as they see fit. Then you practice, practice, practice, because only through using your knowledge will it become readily accessible. Time is finite, and if you want to become immortal you have to live densely, making the best use of what you have to achieve the greatest ends. There is no room for laziness or aimlessness in education, because ultimately you're responsible for all your results, and accepting anything but success means you're fooling yourself.

UNCONVENTIONAL TRAINING

If you walk into any neighborhood globo-gym, what you will find is conventional training. This is true by definition because it's the norm. It's average. Everybody does it. Consequently, when you walk into that globo-gym there's a reason everyone looks and performs at the same level. With the exception of a few genetic lottery-winners and some people that live beneath a squat rack, if you do the same cookie-cutter exercises with the same middling effort, you're going to consistently get the same (lacking) results.

There are plenty of reasons everyone does the same movements. The biggest is that right off the bat when you start something new you follow the crowd. Nobody wants to stand out, at least not in a bad way. And besides, that many people can't be wrong, right?

To step outside the box not only requires courage but consideration. Creative training modalities don't just spring out of thin air. Someone has to invent the tools, understand the math, and build a curriculum around them. Then they have to stick with it through years of trial and error to ensure that what they're doing really works.

Viking Ninja thrives on all things unconventional. We

strive to be exceptional, not ordinary. There are three pillars to this philosophy. The first is unconventional fitness training. That means utilizing tools like the mace or steel clubs to work the body in unique, functional patterns that will translate to real life far better than exercise machines ever could. Second is unconventional recovery modalities. Since few people, if any, actually spend time in active recovery, this box is much easier to check, and it contains all manner of mobility and myofascial release work. Last on the list comes unconventional weapons training, where we utilize timeless tools of the martial arts to improve the connection between mind and body.

Unconventional weapons training is likely the least familiar to most people, as it's rare to find someone who works with eskrima, the bo staff, or other tools like that in the first place. And if you were to use weapons in a dojo, you would probably be training for the purpose of combat or competition. That would be the traditional attitude.

In Viking Ninja, however, we're not aiming for combat. That's not to say tradition is unimportant—tradition is everything—but in this situation our goal is fitness and awakening the Warrior Spirit. More than anything else, it's best looked at as cross-training. Don't get me wrong, weapons work remains martial arts, yet rather than perfecting the skills in their own right, the ultimate goal is to improve your overall coordination and conditioning. For example, it's unlikely in this day and age that you're going to carry nunchucks with you when you go out at night to protect yourself, and it may well be illegal. Yet training with nunchucks will drastically improve your coordination and upper-body strength so that when you get knocked over by some jerk at the nightclub you'll keep from spraining your wrists when you hit the floor, and you'll have the courage to get up and strike back.

Cross-training is aimed at preparing your body for the activities you do regularly. It's about sealing off the weak points in your system to ensure your Yin Yang is balanced. Weapons training provides a type of movement you won't experience in any other activity. As with the steel mace, you're often working with an off-set, levered tool that will challenge your stability and dexterity.

Though we use our hands all day long, we rarely challenge them. They type, they open candy bar wrappers, they pick our noses. But no longer do we climb rough trees, work with hammers and anvils, carve stone weapons, or carry around heavy swords. The hands have tremendous room for improvement, and unconventional weapons training works them in every way. When you get older you don't want to have weak, arthritic fingers that are totally useless. You want a handshake that shows everyone you're still a force to be reckoned with.

Yet it's not just your hands. Your whole body will learn to move differently. Challenging your stability will force you to build untapped supporting musculature. A thousand years ago if you swung a mace or sword and lacked balance, the weight would send you careening off with it. That's when your throat was cut or your knees bashed in. Weapons training teaches you to move in every direction under all conditions.

I don't want you to get in fights. That's not the Viking Ninja way. I do want you to be able to protect yourself, but that's not the point either. Chances are you spend eight hours or more each day in a chair, and consequently you can't move. I want you to be able to move like Muhammad Ali. I want your balance on point. I want your coordination to be lightning fast, your reflexes seamless.

The nunchucks are my favorite tool in our arsenal. Ever since I was a kid watching the Ninja Turtles I knew I was going to master them one day. They're certainly more esoteric than striking, kettlebell training, or anything else you find in your average gym.

You're working with two long, solid handles held together by a heavy chain. It's way different from any other implement in the gym because it's inherently so unstable. The gym is unrealistic, because although it can certainly be dangerous, everything is designed to be as safe and predictable as possible. The real world isn't like that. Real objects are unsteady. You can never expect to have perfect control over anything. Movement is awkward.

When you're swinging nunchucks you always have to be aware that the tool has a mind of its own. That chain changes things dynamically. You're forced to put a hundred percent of your focus into your hands to remove any element of chance you can, and that connection will strengthen the more you play with the tool.

It also challenges your ego. If you look online, you'll find videos of people showing off, yet they only use their right hands. They're not challenging their discipline. With me you're going to work both sides until they're equally skilled. We're not trying to be sexy. We're aiming for skill and self-improvement.

Maybe they're not for everybody, though they would certainly benefit them. What's fascinating to me about teaching nunchucks is that even though they have an unconventional purpose in this system because it's fitness-oriented, I can teach them as if I were running a traditional martial arts school. That's how perfect the tool already is. In a few years they're going to be everywhere.

The bo staff is fitness-oriented as well, yet there's also a tremendous element of creative expression involved. The purpose isn't to dance with the tool, but when you're moving mindfully it can certainly feel and appear that way, considering the rotation and complex footwork. The goal is to apply your body in novel ways. The more variety of movement you go through, the better you adapt to new situations. The ability to learn is itself a learned skill. You begin to see the same patterns in all things, whether it's movement, rote knowledge, or dealing with people better in your life.

With every tool you use, every movement you practice, you must have purpose. I didn't build this system aimlessly. There is always a goal in mind. Unconventional training takes the inherently asymmetrical human body and gives it balance. Symmetry is beautiful, and we stress it through our mindful mechanics, where we mirror movement on each side to shore up weaknesses.

Bruce Lee was always my inspiration. When I was a kid I wanted to be him, but as I got older I realized his path was not my path. I had to do my own thing. Still, his theories had a huge impact on who I am today and what Viking Ninja has become. Bruce Lee argued against blindly following rules. He said to break the system, to take what worked and throw away what didn't. My aim with the nunchucks, the bo staff, striking, recovery, fitness, and everything, really, was to avoid perpetuating the status quo. I wanted to improve upon it and make something new. I want people to break the mold, to learn the tools and then make them their own, not to just find themselves in a new version of the globo-gym where they're all doing the same thing over and over like carbon copies.

Weapons training isn't the first thing that comes to most peoples' minds when they think about fitness. But it doesn't matter who you are, whether you're an athlete or a weekend warrior. We all need focus. We all need to demonstrate to ourselves that we can commit to a physical practice. With these tools and their inherent difficulty comes a reminder of the need for humility, which is the ego's death blow.

And with that comes patience. If you slap yourself on the wrist with your nunchucks, don't shout and throw them at the wall. Each slap should be a reminder that you're the one who controls the tool as well as your emotions. All responsibility lies with you, and losing your temper doesn't help anyone. Take ownership of your actions. No matter what you're doing in life, whether it's cooking, sex, or meditation, this training will teach you how to slow down and get out of your head.

VIKING SHIP ON THE WATER

Imagine the sea, drawn as a child might: a single, waving line across a piece of paper. It can even be blue. And then, upon the water, picture a simple ship. This is one of my favorite teaching tools for Viking Ninja philosophy. It's a fantastic metaphor, and as with everything else, its potential interpretations are limitless.

The ship is full of energy. It's strong, durable, and ready for anything the sea can throw at it. The ship was built for combat. It was built to sail across the sea. And the ship carries Vikings to their destination, where they will conquer. You can also imagine the ship full of ninjas, which is an interesting image to consider because then you have the merging of Viking and Ninja, of Yin and Yang. They too sail across the sea to execute. Ninjas assassinated, while Vikings just wanted something of their own.

Life is water, and water is life. The ship needs water or else it's useless. The Vikings and ninjas that ride in it give the ship direction. But the ocean is intimidating. Open water has driven sailors crazy since the dawn of time. It's just like Bruce Lee's quote. Something as calm as the sea can still destroy you. When you're confronted with something like that, it all comes down to mindset. Are you going to relax or panic? The sea won't kill you—your mindset determines life or death.

Yet sometimes there are storms. The Vikings and ninjas have to be prepared at all times because their lives are on the line. Water is weightless, and so is life. Water can mold around you or it can crush you. Don't be content just because the water's still. You can't grow lazy. That's how you end up capsizing when the first wave comes your way. You'll get smashed against the rocks if you don't pay attention.

Remember, the water represents life. Sometimes it's easy, sometimes it's hard. But if it's easy you can't just sit there treading, because that means you're not exceeding your limits. Life won't deliver for you every time. There are moments for sitting back and enjoying the fruits of your labor, but those are rare occasions to be savored. The Vikings didn't get in that ship for a pleasure ride. They got in there to go somewhere, to conquer, not to grow lazy and fat. They had families to provide for and legends to weave. Even when the water is still you must be hungry.

The water can also be wishy-washy, turbulent, and send you in a variety of directions. Rocking back and forth can make you ill. Life is suffering. Sometimes you'll adapt, but other times you'll just have to keep fighting. What makes this possible is remembering the end goal. You can't get distracted and forget why you're on-board in the first place. That's what makes you go crazy and jump over the rails.

No matter what happens in the water you have to keep a cool head. Did you really expect to sail halfway across the world and not encounter a few waves? Some unsettled seas? This is what the Vikings spent their lives preparing for. You have to trust in your training and keep one eye on the past and the other on the future. Don't forget where you're going or where you came from.

Finally there's the possibility of all-out havoc. There are crashing waves, tumultuous storms, rocks shooting up everywhere. This is where life tries to take you out, where anything that could possibly go wrong rushes in at you from every direction. And this is where the strong are separated from the weak. This is where those with the Warrior Spirit thrive, while those who don't get culled from the herd.

When everything seems to be collapsing inward you turn your game on. When the storms start blowing, the ship must be accountable for itself. The ship is built of durable wood to withstand the elements, and it has an able crew. It's holding us, after all. We trusted the ship to carry us, and our responsibility is to guide the way. We're going to survive. Once we reach land we jump out, execute, and emerge victorious.

Then what? We don't sit on our butts. We don't lounge on the beach we just took with force of arms. We jump on the ship, sail right back into the eye of the storm, and then come out the other side for another battle, another war, ready to conquer again. The great, the powerful, the reliable, they don't fear anything but themselves. And once they've mastered themselves, there's nothing left in their way.

The Viking ship also represents community. There are seats for twenty, fifty, a hundred down in the galley. One man can't propel a whole ship across the sea. It's designed to hold a brotherhood, a sisterhood, any and everybody that's willing to pitch in. All the passengers have the same goal, and they're in that ship for one reason. They want to survive the voyage and reap the rewards of whatever's on the other side.

The ship holds family bound by honor, and family sticks together. One person doesn't make an army. One person can't get anywhere. How do they pump a hundred oars while manning the wheel? Folding and unfurling the sail? It's impossible. They sink way before the storm ever arrives. They can't even handle the calm seas. That ship's going to spring leaks and two hands can't bail out all the water before it sinks. There's no Vegvisir Compass, no center. You're bound to fail if you go it alone. We all need a crew, even if it's just for support.

The ship is made of the purest Norwegian wood. It's made of heart, it's made of soul, it's made of commitment. If the community is united, nothing can break those bonds. It won't spring leaks. The more people that are part of the community, that contribute their energy and passion to the ship, the stronger it gets. If one person has to get off the oars, another person will be more than happy to take their place. In storms you'll have twenty people bailing water and another twenty waiting to take over the moment they get tired.

Any time you set out to sea you're taking a stand. You're addressing a challenge and saying you can handle it. Trees aren't meant to survive on water. They're born of the earth in dirt. The ship dares the water to wreck it, but in the process land and water become unified. They find balance through the Yin Yang. The solid and the formless work as one. Even though passion rages and the sea is wild, they stay together and get you to the other side. When your energy resonates with the challenges you face, when there's perfect symmetry and synchronicity and flow, that's when you find your most powerful, optimized self.

And where's the ship's destination? It's just like the Vegvisir Compass. Wherever you go, wherever you land—that's the destination. As long as you're following your path, as long as you're true to your mind and body, you're going in the right direction. All you have to do is own it. You don't have to land in any particular place. We're all going somewhere unique, though if we're part of a community we may head in a similar direction.

It's important that the ship you ride in be strong. Your organization, your brotherhood—whatever it is—must be built on a strong foundation. You can't just gather your people and hop in a little buoy boat to cross the ocean. It may get you across a pond, but if you have serious ambitions you need a serious ship. As soon as you hit turbulence the boat will break and you'll all drown.

You need stability, honesty, truth. Big waves rock a small craft. Be careful who you take aboard with you, because when you're stuck in the middle of the ocean you can't change ships or people. The best thing to do is be careful before you push off. Otherwise you might end up shipwrecked and without even a sturdy plank to hang onto.

I also like to imagine the ship not as a community, but as a metaphor for the individual. If you are the ship, then the water is your mind. The Valknut is by nature turbulent, yet to get from point A to B you must find balance. You have to calm the water, and that means centering yourself through the Yin Yang.

When you're the ship, understand that you come from land. You're in foreign territory, and you need to make the most of it. You're riding a wave. You can't control it, but you can do your best to hold on. Ultimately the weather, the rain, lightning—it's out of our control. All we can do is prepare as best we can, make the proper choices beforehand, and keep our intentions pure when we hit the water.

AFTERWORD

Though the seed was conceived when I was much younger, Viking Ninja was born during my time at Onnit. Total Human Optimization—linking the mind, body, and spirit to create something amazing—inspired me. Hopefully after reading this book you understand how Viking Ninja seeks the same. All three elements of a person are connected, and without devoting them equal attention you will be imbalanced. As a fitness system, we use the body to push ourselves mentally and spiritually, so that while we improve physically we simultaneously develop our other two primary components.

The first part of our motto is, "Kill your ego." It's impossible to reach Total Human Optimization or access your Warrior Spirit if you neglect this key part of the equation. Integral to improvement is growth, but you can't grow if you aren't open to it. Ego in this sense equates to overbearing pride and arrogance. If you approach a teacher, attend a class, or enter your gym with the belief that you know all the answers, there won't be room to increase your knowledge.

The second part of our motto is, "Challenge your discipline." The simple fact of the matter is that we will never get anywhere if we don't apply ourselves to the fullest extent of our abilities. The key word here is *apply*. Shutting down the ego is only the first step. So, you're not the end-all be-all of your existence. What now? You get to work. This means picking up a steel mace and doing 360s until your hands ache. It means reading a book like this. It means flexing your muscles—physical, mental, and spiritual—until you've surpassed yourself.

As far as I'm concerned, you can't read this quote from Bruce Lee often enough, so here's another dose:

> "You might as well be dead. Seriously, if you always put limits on what you can do, physically or anything else, it'll spread over into the rest of your life. It'll spread into your work, into your morality, into your entire being. There are no limits. There are plateaus, but you must not stay there, you must go beyond them. If it kills you, it kills you. A man must constantly exceed his level."

This is why I wrote the book you're holding right now. It's the reason I started Viking Ninja. Why live, why do anything in the first place, if our goal isn't to experience life to the fullest?

If you're on the jiu-jitsu mats, your aim isn't to get submitted the same way every day, never learning anything. There's no fun in that. It's the same with tennis, writing, cooking, or anything else. There's more to life than the average, the just-barely-adequate, and it's your responsibility to press through that.

The natural state of anything is inertia. It makes no difference whether you're a person or a bowling ball. And that's what setting limitations does. It stops you from moving forward. Bruce Lee was right when he said there are no limits. Each hour you can learn something new, try harder at what you already do, or in some other way explore the infinitude of possibility waiting you.

Pivotal to this enterprise is open-mindedness. Again, consider Bruce Lee, though this time the idea of the empty cup. If you go to jiu-jitsu class (or astronomy, dance, or carpentry) and are unwilling to apply yourself, how will you benefit? At least on the mats you can expect to be choked out if you don't internalize the principles. There's a time for self-expression in any art, but before that comes mastery of the basics. There's no better advice than learning to walk before you run, and if you're adamantly opposed to walking you'll never be able to sprint, jump, or skip.

You must also tap into your Warrior Spirit, another thing Bruce Lee knew more than a little about. The simple desire to improve yourself is insufficient. Everybody wants to be exceptional, but few of us ever achieve it. By definition the majority of people are either average or below it. Am I okay with being an average saxophonist? Yes, and that's okay. It's not my priority. Yet if fitness is my life and something I care deeply about, I can't accept the average.

My duty is to wake up every morning aiming to be the best in the world at what I do. This attitude isn't bred by complacency, but the tenacity of the Warrior Spirit. Countless people want to write or swing the mace, yet they twiddle their thumbs instead because it's easier. Kindle within you the fire to act and never let it go out.

One of the most crucial aspects of Viking Ninja to grasp is that you are not alone. We're a community, and together we stand strong. We share values, and negativity isn't tolerated. If we were on a Viking ship, the people who wouldn't row, who lie and steal, would be thrown overboard. Everyone here wants to help you, and your duty is to help them back. We are far more resilient, far more effective, when we work together than when we toil alone.

If you live in the middle of nowhere it will be a lot easier to swing the mace every day if you have a group of friends who push each other to do the same. No matter how fancy your gear is, it's impossible to spar alone. Having people to learn from brings you new knowledge, while teaching allows you to concretize whatever material it is you're sharing. Never cast away a friend who's willing to watch your back. In the quest for optimization that can mean life or death, success or failure.

Seize every minute of every day. Juice each opportunity for what it's worth. This means spending countless hours practicing, but it also means searching for fresh education whenever possible. The people who came before you in any given pursuit have been through the same journey you're about to undertake, yet you have the advantage in that they've already processed and refined the lessons they learned. If someone is willing to share that, you can cut down on the time it will take to achieve any given level of proficiency in your area of interest. Never refuse help out of pride from someone who can lift you to a higher order of existence.

I hope we succeeded in sharing with you the core tenets of Viking Ninja philosophy in a clear and sensical way. Now your task is to consider it for yourself and determine whether you share our values. The rabbit hole goes deep, and there will certainly be more, but these chapters form the basis of the system.

When I look at the Valknut it's likely that I see something completely different from what you see. Just as we are all unique, we perceive the world as individuals. No one's viewpoint is less valuable than another's. What matters is how they serve you. As long as you find inspiration and value in the symbols, concepts, and philosophy, then they are meaningful.

Take what you learn and integrate it into your life. Otherwise the material is worthless. I can't tell you how many books I've read, been inspired by, and then completely forgotten, failing to implement even the most basic principles. Don't let that happen to you. It stunts your growth. Read the book again if you have to, taking notes on how you can use the philosophy in daily life. Commit to it.

Though we begin our training with the body, everything is mental. Whether that's stopping halfway through a round of Viking Striking or setting limits on what you can achieve, your mind makes the decision. Your mind and spirit control the body—nothing else. The heart beats, the lungs breathe, but your arms and legs don't act of their own accord. Your job is to strengthen your will to the greatest extent possible, eliminating fear, weakness, ego, and anything else that could possibly sabotage you. This is where symbols and philosophy become so powerful—they're a constant reminder of your values and potential.

That's not to say the physical element is unimportant. It's necessary, but worthless if your mind isn't engaged. The dependence works both ways. A book can teach you a lot, yet you can't learn how to wield the steel mace without swinging it, nor can you become a champion UFC fighter without ever throwing a punch. While this text is full of abstract material, to succeed in the system you must seek out physical instruction, whether that means attending certifications and workshops or simply finding videos and articles to push you in the right direction.

Buy yourself a steel mace. They're cheap. Start swinging it. Write about your life. Where do you want to be? What do you want to do? What's keeping you from getting there? If you don't have a community that values what you do and is actively helping you reach your dreams, then find people who will support you. I can think of at least one group that's readily available and willing to be part of your life. Delve deep into movement. Spend time pondering your innermost feelings and desires. Nurture the spirit. Kill your ego and challenge your discipline.

Awaken the warrior within.

If you haven't yet, please consider leaving a review on Amazon. For a book like this, every last one counts and helps us reach more people with our message.

Sign up for our newsletter to learn more about the Viking Ninja belting system, training, and events at VKNJA.com.

Check out Erik Melland on Instagram at @erikmelland. For more ideas and inspiration, follow @VKNJA.

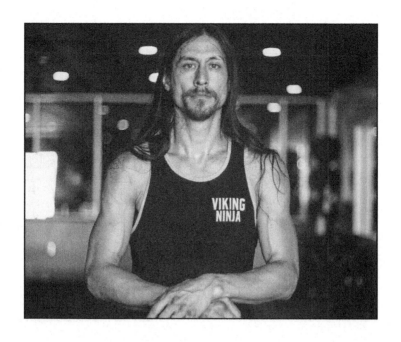

Erik Melland

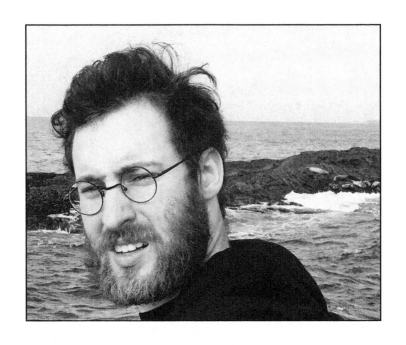

Robinson Erhardt

Made in the USA
Las Vegas, NV
19 February 2021